UNDERSTANDING WEIGHT MANAGEMENT: 2024 EDITION

BY:

MARK BARNETT

Introduction

In an era characterized by rapid technological advancements and an evolving understanding of health and wellness, the quest for effective weight management has taken center stage in the pursuit of a healthier lifestyle. "UNDERSTANDING WEIGHT MANAGEMENT: 2024 EDITION" is a comprehensive guide that navigates the landscape of modern weight control methods, shedding light on innovative approaches and emerging trends reshaping the way we perceive and achieve optimal health.

This book ventures beyond traditional notions of dieting and exercise, delving into the dynamic realm of cutting-edge technologies, personalized strategies, and holistic approaches that redefine the paradigms of weight management. With a fusion of scientific insights, practical advice, and forward-thinking concepts, this guide aims to empower individuals seeking sustainable and personalized solutions for achieving and maintaining a healthy weight.

Within these pages, readers will embark on an enlightening journey through the latest advancements in wearable technology, artificial intelligence, personalized nutrition, behavioral sciences, and holistic wellness practices. From the impact of wearable devices in tracking physical activity to the profound implications of AI-driven personalized nutrition, each chapter unveils the transformative potential of these innovations in sculpting a healthier and more balanced life.

Moreover, this book transcends mere technological marvels, encompassing the significance of social support networks, mental well-being, and the intricate interplay between genetics, environment, and lifestyle choices in the realm of weight management. It illuminates the role of family, friends,

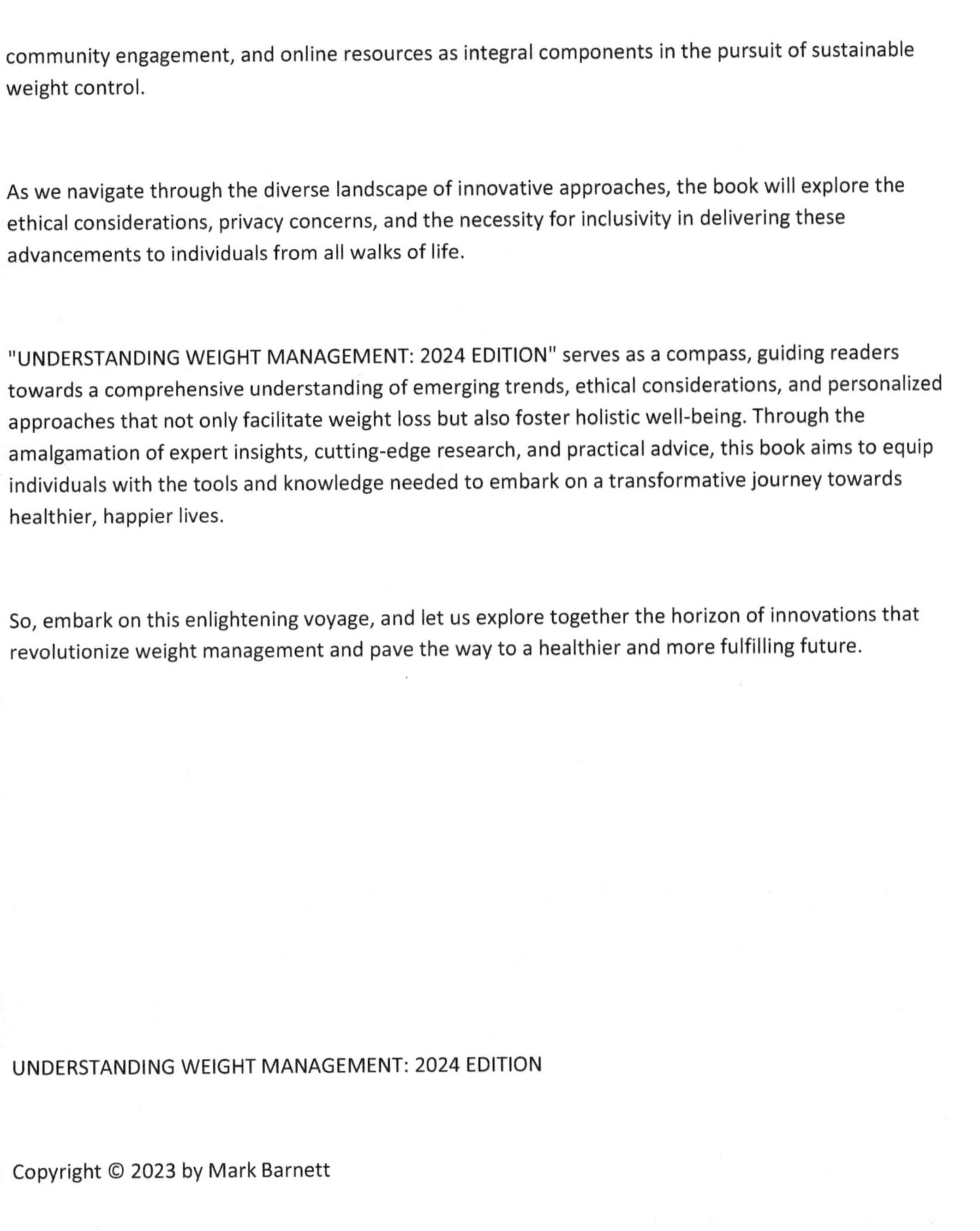

community engagement, and online resources as integral components in the pursuit of sustainable weight control.

As we navigate through the diverse landscape of innovative approaches, the book will explore the ethical considerations, privacy concerns, and the necessity for inclusivity in delivering these advancements to individuals from all walks of life.

"UNDERSTANDING WEIGHT MANAGEMENT: 2024 EDITION" serves as a compass, guiding readers towards a comprehensive understanding of emerging trends, ethical considerations, and personalized approaches that not only facilitate weight loss but also foster holistic well-being. Through the amalgamation of expert insights, cutting-edge research, and practical advice, this book aims to equip individuals with the tools and knowledge needed to embark on a transformative journey towards healthier, happier lives.

So, embark on this enlightening voyage, and let us explore together the horizon of innovations that revolutionize weight management and pave the way to a healthier and more fulfilling future.

UNDERSTANDING WEIGHT MANAGEMENT: 2024 EDITION

Published by: Mark Barnett

Cover Design by: Mark Barnett

Printed in: United States of America (USA)

UNDERSTANDING WEIGHT MANAGEMENT: 2024 EDITION

CHAPTER 1

Weight management is a multifaceted and evolving discipline that transcends mere numbers on a scale. In contemporary society, the pursuit of healthy weight and body composition encompasses a blend of scientific understanding, individualized approaches, behavioral modifications, and societal influences. This introduction aims to elucidate the evolving landscape of weight management, encapsulating its multidimensional nature and the innovative methodologies that underpin its modern interpretation.

The Changing Paradigm of Weight Management

The traditional notion of weight management often fixated on caloric restriction and increased physical activity as the primary means to achieve weight-related goals. However, the paradigm has shifted, acknowledging the intricate interplay between genetics, metabolism, environment, psychological factors, and lifestyle choices in determining an individual's weight status.

Holistic Perspective: Modern weight management adopts a holistic perspective, recognizing that successful and sustainable weight control extends beyond dietary modifications and exercise regimens. It encompasses mental well-being, sleep patterns, stress management, gut health, hormonal balance, social support structures, and overall lifestyle choices.

Individualized Approach: There is no one-size-fits-all solution in modern weight management. Recognizing the uniqueness of each individual's physiology, preferences, and challenges has spurred a shift toward personalized strategies. Tailoring interventions based on genetic predispositions, metabolic profiles, and behavioral tendencies is gaining prominence.

The Science Behind Weight Regulation

Understanding the science of weight regulation forms the cornerstone of modern weight management approaches. Metabolism, hormonal influences, genetic predispositions, and environmental factors intricately govern an individual's weight.

Metabolism: Metabolism, often misconstrued as solely pertaining to the rate at which the body burns calories, is a complex process involving numerous biochemical reactions. Basal metabolic rate (BMR), thermic effect of food (TEF), and physical activity thermogenesis (PAT) collectively determine an individual's energy expenditure.

Genetics and Environment: Genetic factors predispose individuals to different metabolic rates, fat storage tendencies, and responses to dietary and exercise interventions. However, environmental influences, including diet, physical activity levels, socio-economic status, and access to healthy foods, play a pivotal role in shaping weight outcomes.

Hormonal Regulation: Hormones intricately regulate hunger, satiety, and energy balance. Leptin, ghrelin, insulin, cortisol, and other hormones influence appetite, metabolism, and fat storage, contributing significantly to weight regulation.

Embracing a Holistic Lifestyle Approach

Modern weight management acknowledges that achieving and maintaining a healthy weight involves embracing a lifestyle that fosters overall well-being.

Nutrition Strategies: Beyond calorie counting, emphasis is placed on the quality of food consumed. Balanced macronutrient intake, micronutrient sufficiency, mindful eating practices, and tailored dietary plans based on individual needs form the crux of nutrition strategies.

Physical Activity: Exercise is not merely a tool for burning calories; it is a means to improve cardiovascular health, build lean muscle mass, enhance metabolism, and promote mental well-being. Diverse exercise modalities, including strength training, cardio, flexibility, and functional training, cater to varied fitness goals.

Mental Health and Stress Management: Acknowledging the profound impact of psychological well-being on weight, strategies encompass stress reduction techniques, cognitive behavioral therapy (CBT), mindfulness practices, and fostering a positive body image.

Sleep Optimization: The intricate link between sleep patterns and weight regulation is increasingly recognized. Prioritizing adequate and quality sleep supports hormonal balance, appetite regulation, and overall metabolic health.

Integrating Technology and Innovations

Advancements in technology have revolutionized the landscape of weight management, offering innovative tools and solutions to aid individuals in their journey toward better health.

Wearable Devices: From fitness trackers to smart scales and apps, wearable technology provides real-time data on physical activity, sleep patterns, calorie expenditure, and even stress levels, enabling individuals to make informed decisions.

AI and Personalized Solutions: Artificial intelligence (AI) and machine learning algorithms analyze vast datasets to offer personalized recommendations on nutrition, exercise routines, and behavioral modifications tailored to an individual's goals and preferences.

Online Communities and Support Systems: Virtual communities, social media platforms, and online forums serve as invaluable resources, fostering support, sharing experiences, and providing guidance in navigating the challenges of weight management.

Defining Modern Perspectives on Weight Management

1.2 Importance of a Holistic Approach

In the landscape of modern weight management, a paradigm shift has occurred, pivoting from the conventional focus solely on diet and exercise to a more comprehensive, holistic approach. This shift is rooted in acknowledging that weight management extends far beyond mere physical interventions. A holistic perspective recognizes the intricate interplay of various factors contributing to an individual's weight status and overall well-being.

Multidimensional Nature of Weight Management: Holistic weight management acknowledges that an individual's weight is influenced by a multitude of factors, including genetics, metabolism, hormonal balance, psychological well-being, lifestyle choices, social environment, and even cultural influences. These elements collectively shape an individual's relationship with food, physical activity, and body image.

Mental and Emotional Well-being: Recognizing the intimate connection between mental health and weight, modern approaches to weight management emphasize addressing emotional eating patterns, stress management, body image issues, and fostering a positive mindset. Techniques like mindfulness, cognitive behavioral therapy (CBT), and stress reduction strategies are integrated to promote a healthy relationship with food and self-image.

Lifestyle Modifications: Holistic weight management extends beyond short-term fixes; it revolves around sustainable lifestyle modifications. It emphasizes the importance of sleep optimization, healthy eating habits, regular physical activity, and managing daily stressors as integral components of achieving and maintaining a healthy weight.

Individualized Strategies: Embracing a holistic approach involves recognizing that each person's journey towards weight management is unique. Personalized strategies tailored to an individual's preferences, genetics, metabolic profile, and socio-environmental factors are vital for long-term success.

1.3 Overview of the Book's Structure

This book serves as a comprehensive guide to modern weight management, structured to provide a nuanced understanding of diverse aspects crucial for achieving sustainable weight control and overall well-being. Here is an overview of the book's structure, delineating the chapters and their core focuses:

Part 1: Understanding Weight Management

Chapter 1: Introduction to Modern Weight Management

Provides an overview of the evolving landscape of weight management and the transition towards holistic approaches.

Emphasizes the multidimensional nature of weight control and its broader implications on health and well-being.

Chapter 2: The Science of Weight Loss and Gain

Explores the scientific underpinnings of weight regulation, encompassing metabolism, genetics, hormonal influences, and environmental factors.

Discusses how these factors interplay to influence an individual's weight status.

Part 2: Nutrition Strategies for Weight Management

Chapter 3: Macro and Micro-Nutrients

Examines the significance of macronutrients and micronutrients in supporting weight management goals.

Provides insights into creating balanced meals and dietary plans for effective weight control.

Chapter 4: Innovative Diets for Weight Control

Explores emerging and innovative dietary approaches, such as intermittent fasting, plant-based diets, and their impact on weight management.

Evaluates the effectiveness and customization of different diet plans for diverse lifestyles.

Part 3: Exercise and Physical Activity

Chapter 5: Exercise and Weight Loss

Discusses the role of various exercise modalities in weight management, including high-intensity interval training (HIIT), resistance training, and cardio exercises.

Explores how exercise influences metabolism, muscle mass, and overall weight regulation.

Chapter 6: Non-Traditional Approaches to Fitness

Explores alternative exercise forms like yoga, Pilates, and mind-body practices in weight management.

Highlights the integration of technology and outdoor activities in promoting physical activity for weight control.

Part 4: Lifestyle Changes for Weight Maintenance

Chapter 7: Sleep and Weight Management

Examines the correlation between sleep patterns and weight regulation.

Provides strategies for improving sleep quality to support weight control.

Chapter 8: Stress Management and Weight

Explores the impact of stress on weight gain and strategies to mitigate stress for better weight management outcomes.

Discusses the importance of mindfulness and mental health practices.

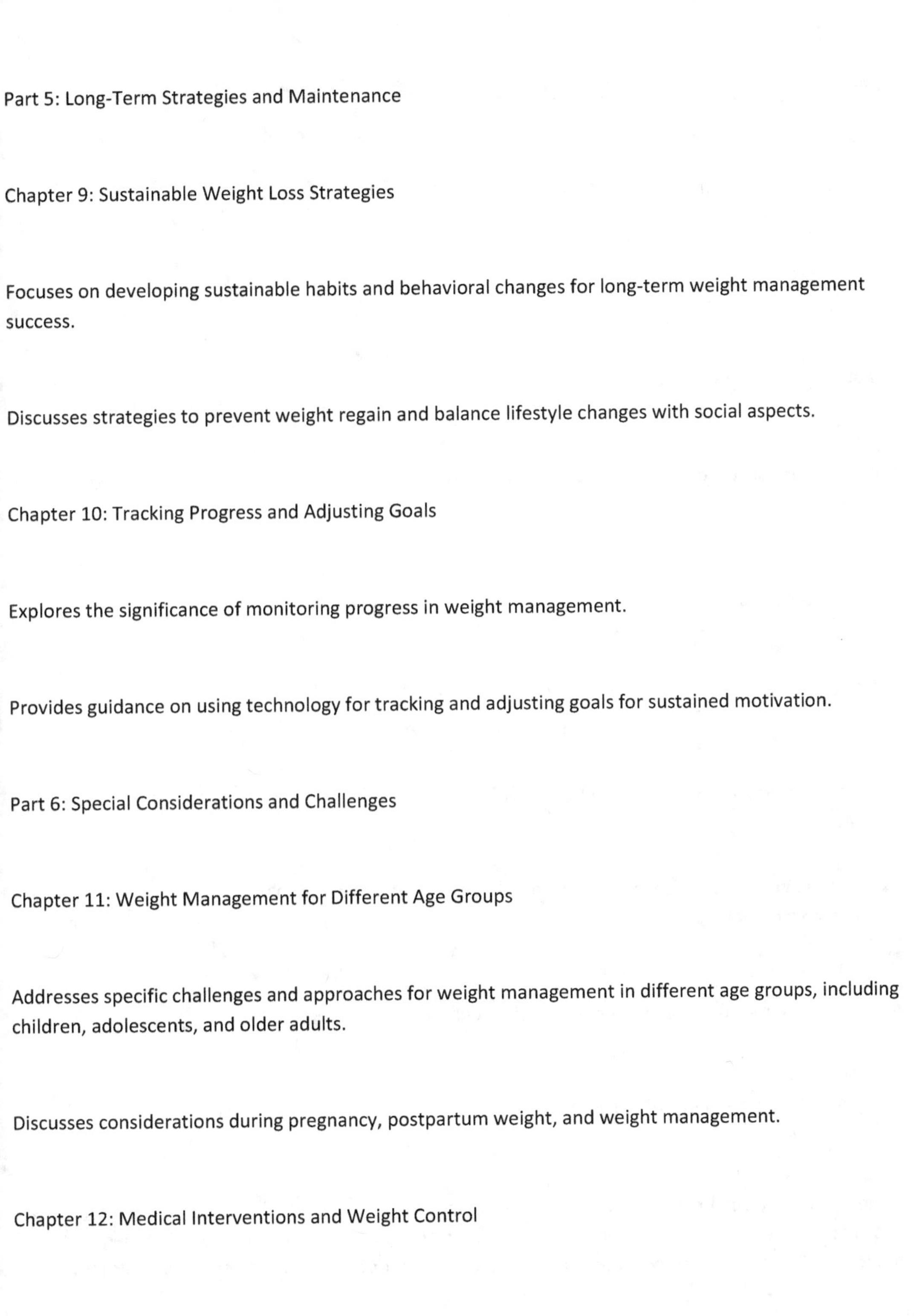

Part 5: Long-Term Strategies and Maintenance

Chapter 9: Sustainable Weight Loss Strategies

Focuses on developing sustainable habits and behavioral changes for long-term weight management success.

Discusses strategies to prevent weight regain and balance lifestyle changes with social aspects.

Chapter 10: Tracking Progress and Adjusting Goals

Explores the significance of monitoring progress in weight management.

Provides guidance on using technology for tracking and adjusting goals for sustained motivation.

Part 6: Special Considerations and Challenges

Chapter 11: Weight Management for Different Age Groups

Addresses specific challenges and approaches for weight management in different age groups, including children, adolescents, and older adults.

Discusses considerations during pregnancy, postpartum weight, and weight management.

Chapter 12: Medical Interventions and Weight Control

Explores medical options, including bariatric surgery, medications, and their role in weight management.

Discusses the pros, cons, and considerations for medical interventions.

Part 7: Social Support and Community Engagement

Chapter 13: Importance of Support Systems

Highlights the role of social support structures, family, friends, and online communities in weight management.

Discusses the impact of community engagement on motivation and accountability.

Part 8: Future Trends and Innovations

Chapter 14: Emerging Technologies in Weight Management

Explores the integration of technology, wearable devices, AI, and personalized solutions in modern weight management.

Predicts future trends and advancements in the field.

The Science of Weight Loss and Gain

Understanding the complex interplay of factors that govern weight loss and gain involves delving into the multifaceted realm of human metabolism, genetics, hormonal regulation, and environmental influences. This comprehensive understanding forms the bedrock of effective and sustainable strategies in modern weight management.

Metabolism and Energy Balance

Metabolism: Metabolism is the culmination of biochemical processes that occur within the body to sustain life. At its core, it involves converting food into energy, which the body utilizes for various functions, including basal metabolic rate (BMR), physical activity, and the thermic effect of food (TEF).

Energy Balance: Weight management is intricately tied to the concept of energy balance, which is the relationship between the energy consumed through food and beverages and the energy expended through metabolic processes and physical activity. A negative energy balance results in weight loss, while a positive energy balance leads to weight gain.

Genetic Predisposition and Environmental Influences

Genetics: Genetic predispositions significantly influence an individual's propensity for weight gain or loss. Variations in genes related to metabolism, fat storage, appetite regulation, and hormonal responses to food impact how the body processes nutrients and manages weight.

Environmental Factors: Beyond genetics, environmental influences play a crucial role in weight regulation. Socio-economic status, access to nutritious foods, cultural dietary habits, built environments that support physical activity, and stress levels are among the myriad external factors that shape an individual's weight status.

Hormonal Regulation and Appetite Control

Leptin and Ghrelin: Hormones such as leptin and ghrelin are key players in regulating hunger and satiety. Leptin, often referred to as the "satiety hormone," signals fullness to the brain, suppressing appetite. Ghrelin, conversely known as the "hunger hormone," stimulates appetite, prompting food intake.

Insulin and Blood Sugar: Insulin, produced by the pancreas, regulates blood sugar levels and facilitates the storage of excess glucose as fat. Imbalances in insulin levels can lead to weight gain and metabolic disorders like insulin resistance.

Understanding Weight Loss Strategies

Caloric Deficit: The cornerstone of weight loss remains achieving a caloric deficit, where the body expends more energy than it consumes. This deficit can be attained through dietary changes, increased physical activity, or a combination of both.

Macronutrient Balance: While calorie control is vital, the quality of nutrients consumed also matters. Balancing macronutrients—proteins, carbohydrates, and fats—ensures adequate energy levels, muscle preservation, and satiety.

Metabolic Adaptation: The body tends to adapt to reduced calorie intake by slowing metabolism to conserve energy, making weight loss more challenging over time. Strategies to counteract this adaptation involve periodic refeeding or adjusting caloric intake.

Weight Gain Factors

Energy Surplus: Weight gain occurs when the body consistently consumes more calories than it expends. Excessive calorie intake, often coupled with a sedentary lifestyle, leads to the storage of excess energy as fat.

Unhealthy Eating Patterns: Poor dietary choices, including high-calorie processed foods, sugary beverages, and excessive consumption of refined carbohydrates, contribute to weight gain. These foods often lack essential nutrients and promote overeating due to their low satiety value.

Sedentary Lifestyle: Physical inactivity is a significant contributor to weight gain. A lack of regular exercise diminishes energy expenditure, leading to the accumulation of excess body fat and a decline in overall metabolic health.

Environmental and Societal Impacts on Weight Regulation

Food Environment: The modern food environment, characterized by the ubiquity of highly processed, calorie-dense foods, promotes overeating and contributes to weight gain. Additionally, larger portion sizes and easy access to fast food exacerbate this issue.

Societal Norms and Perception: Cultural and societal norms regarding body image, beauty standards, and societal pressure can influence an individual's perception of weight. This can lead to disordered eating patterns, unhealthy weight control behaviors, and psychological stress related to body image.

Strategies for Effective Weight Management

Individualized Approach: Recognizing the uniqueness of each individual's physiology, genetics, and lifestyle, personalized approaches to weight management are crucial for long-term success. Tailoring interventions based on an individual's metabolic profile, preferences, and challenges yields more sustainable outcomes.

Behavioral Changes: Shifting focus from short-term fixes to long-lasting behavioral changes forms the cornerstone of effective weight management. Encouraging healthier eating habits, regular physical activity, stress reduction, and improved sleep patterns fosters sustainable lifestyle modifications.

Comprehensive Lifestyle Modifications: Holistic approaches encompassing nutrition, exercise, stress management, sleep optimization, and psychological well-being are integral in achieving and maintaining a healthy weight. These strategies address various facets of an individual's life, promoting overall health and vitality.

Conclusion

The science behind weight loss and gain is a multifaceted tapestry woven by genetics, metabolism, hormonal regulation, environmental influences, and lifestyle choices. Acknowledging these complexities forms the basis for crafting effective and sustainable strategies in modern weight management. Recognizing the individuality of each person's journey and employing evidence-based approaches encompassing comprehensive lifestyle modifications is paramount in fostering long-term success in weight control and overall well-being. Understanding the intricacies of weight regulation empowers individuals to make informed choices and navigate their path towards a healthier and balanced life.

Understanding Metabolism and its Role in Weight Management

Metabolism: A Complex Mechanism

Metabolism is the intricate process by which the body converts food and beverages into energy. It comprises various biochemical reactions that sustain life by providing the energy necessary for bodily functions, such as breathing, cell repair, digestion, and movement.

Components of Metabolism

Basal Metabolic Rate (BMR): BMR represents the energy the body expends while at rest to maintain vital functions like breathing and cell repair. It accounts for the largest portion of daily energy expenditure, around 60-75% in most individuals.

Thermic Effect of Food (TEF): TEF reflects the energy used to digest, absorb, and process nutrients from food. Different macronutrients have varying TEF rates, with protein requiring the most energy for digestion, followed by carbohydrates and fats.

Physical Activity Thermogenesis (PAT): PAT encompasses the energy expended during physical activity, including exercise, daily chores, and any movement beyond resting metabolic rate.

Role of Metabolism in Weight Management

Metabolism plays a pivotal role in weight management as it determines how efficiently the body utilizes energy. A higher metabolism implies a greater calorie burn, which may facilitate weight loss. However, numerous factors influence metabolic rate, including age, gender, muscle mass, hormone levels, and genetics.

Impact of Genetics and Environment on Weight

Genetics and Weight Predisposition

Genetic Variations: Genetic factors significantly contribute to an individual's predisposition to weight gain or loss. Variations in genes related to metabolism, appetite regulation, fat storage, and energy expenditure can influence susceptibility to obesity.

Heritability of Weight Traits: Studies suggest that genetic factors may account for 40-70% of an individual's weight status. However, genetics do not solely determine weight; they interact with environmental factors in a complex manner.

Environmental Influences on Weight

Dietary Habits: Access to highly processed, calorie-dense foods, coupled with high intake of sugars, unhealthy fats, and low nutrient density, contributes to weight gain.

Physical Activity Levels: Sedentary lifestyles, characterized by limited physical activity and increased screen time, lead to reduced energy expenditure and contribute to weight gain.

Socio-Economic Factors: Socio-economic disparities, including limited access to nutritious foods, food insecurity, and lack of resources for physical activity, contribute to obesity in marginalized populations.

Hormonal Influences on Weight Regulation

Leptin: The Satiety Hormone

Role of Leptin: Leptin, produced by fat cells, signals the brain to regulate appetite and energy balance. Higher levels of leptin typically indicate satiety, signaling the body to reduce food intake and increase energy expenditure.

Leptin Resistance: In some individuals with obesity, despite high leptin levels, the brain doesn't respond effectively to its signals, leading to leptin resistance. This resistance impairs the regulation of appetite and may contribute to weight gain.

Ghrelin: The Hunger Hormone

Ghrelin's Influence: Ghrelin, produced in the stomach, stimulates appetite and promotes food intake. Its levels rise before meals and decrease after eating, signaling hunger and satiety, respectively.

Hormonal Imbalance and Weight: Imbalances in ghrelin levels or sensitivity to its signals can disrupt hunger regulation, potentially contributing to overeating and weight gain.

Interplay of Metabolism, Genetics, Environment, and Hormones in Weight Management

Integrating Factors for Effective Strategies

Individualized Approach: Recognizing the unique interaction of genetics, metabolism, hormonal regulation, and environmental influences is crucial for tailoring effective weight management strategies.

Lifestyle Modifications: Emphasizing comprehensive lifestyle changes encompassing healthy eating habits, regular physical activity, stress reduction, adequate sleep, and mindful choices to mitigate the impact of genetic predispositions and hormonal imbalances on weight.

Personalized Interventions: Using insights from genetics, metabolism, and hormonal profiles to personalize dietary plans, exercise regimens, and behavioral interventions for sustainable weight control.

Conclusion

Understanding metabolism, genetic predispositions, environmental influences, and hormonal regulation provides a holistic perspective on weight management. While genetics and metabolism lay the foundation, environmental factors and hormonal balance significantly influence an individual's weight status. By recognizing and addressing these multifaceted factors, personalized and comprehensive strategies can be devised to facilitate effective weight management, promoting overall health and well-being.

UNDERSTANDING WEIGHT MANAGEMENT: 2024 EDITION

CHAPTER 2

The Psychological Dimensions of Weight Management

Emotional Eating and Stress

Emotional Eating: Emotional triggers such as stress, anxiety, depression, or even joy can influence eating behaviors. Using food as a coping mechanism to manage emotions often leads to overeating or consuming comfort foods high in calories, sugars, or fats.

Stress and Weight: Chronic stress triggers the release of cortisol, a hormone that can stimulate appetite and lead to increased food intake, especially high-calorie foods. This response can contribute to weight gain over time.

Body Image and Self-Esteem

Body Image Disturbance: Poor body image, characterized by dissatisfaction with one's appearance, can lead to disordered eating habits, excessive dieting, and psychological distress, impacting mental health and potentially contributing to weight fluctuations.

Self-Esteem and Weight: Low self-esteem and negative body image often correlate with weight-related issues, affecting an individual's confidence and self-worth. These factors can create barriers to adopting healthy lifestyle changes.

Psychological Factors Influencing Behavior

Mindset and Behavioral Patterns

Mindset and Weight Management: Attitude and beliefs regarding weight management significantly impact behavior. A growth mindset that views setbacks as opportunities for learning and growth promotes resilience in weight management efforts.

Behavioral Patterns: Habits, routines, and learned behaviors significantly influence eating patterns, physical activity levels, and overall lifestyle choices. Identifying and modifying unhealthy behavioral patterns is essential for sustainable weight management.

Stress Management and Coping Strategies

Stress Reduction Techniques

Stress Management: Implementing stress reduction techniques such as mindfulness, meditation, deep breathing exercises, or yoga can mitigate the impact of stress on eating behaviors and help in controlling emotional eating triggers.

Cognitive Behavioral Therapy (CBT): CBT, a therapeutic approach, helps individuals identify and modify negative thought patterns and behaviors related to food, body image, and weight, fostering healthier relationships with food and promoting weight management.

Addressing Mental Health for Effective Weight Management

Holistic Approach to Well-being

Integrated Approach: Recognizing the interplay between mental health, emotional well-being, and weight management, adopting a holistic approach that integrates mental health interventions into weight management strategies is vital.

Professional Support: Seeking guidance from mental health professionals, dietitians, or therapists can provide personalized strategies to address underlying emotional triggers, promote healthier coping mechanisms, and foster positive behavioral changes.

Conclusion

The intricate connection between mental health and weight underscores the importance of addressing psychological well-being in weight management efforts. Emotional eating patterns, stress, body image disturbances, and unhealthy coping mechanisms significantly impact eating behaviors and lifestyle choices, influencing weight outcomes. Employing stress reduction techniques, cognitive behavioral therapy, and adopting a holistic approach to well-being can empower individuals to manage their mental health while making sustainable changes for effective weight management.

Exploring the Psychological Aspects of Weight Management

Addressing Emotional Eating

Understanding Emotional Eating: Emotional eating involves using food as a coping mechanism to manage emotions rather than to satisfy physical hunger. It often stems from stress, anxiety, boredom, or sadness, leading to overconsumption of high-calorie, comfort foods.

Identifying Triggers: Recognizing emotional triggers that prompt unhealthy eating behaviors is pivotal. Stressful situations, negative emotions, or specific events often serve as cues for emotional eating. Awareness is the first step toward addressing this pattern.

Coping Mechanisms: Developing alternative coping mechanisms beyond food is crucial. Engaging in activities such as exercise, journaling, mindfulness practices, or seeking social support can help manage emotions without resorting to emotional eating.

Overcoming Mental Barriers

Self-Limiting Beliefs: Mental barriers, such as negative self-talk, unrealistic expectations, fear of failure, or lack of self-confidence, can impede progress in weight management efforts.

Changing Mindset: Adopting a growth mindset that focuses on progress rather than perfection is essential. Setting realistic goals, celebrating small victories, and reframing setbacks as learning opportunities can help overcome mental barriers.

Seeking Support: Utilizing support systems, including friends, family, or professional guidance, can provide encouragement, accountability, and guidance in navigating mental barriers and fostering a positive mindset.

Strategies for Promoting a Positive Body Image

Understanding Body Image

Body Image Perception: Body image encompasses an individual's perceptions, thoughts, and feelings about their physical appearance. It's shaped by societal standards, cultural influences, media portrayals, and personal experiences.

Impact on Behavior: Poor body image can lead to disordered eating patterns, low self-esteem, and mental health issues. Addressing and fostering a positive body image is crucial for overall well-being.

Cultivating a Positive Body Image

Self-Acceptance and Self-Compassion: Encouraging self-acceptance and self-compassion plays a pivotal role. Embracing one's body and acknowledging its strengths beyond appearance fosters a healthier relationship with oneself.

Healthy Lifestyle Focus: Shifting focus from appearance-based goals to health-oriented objectives promotes a positive body image. Emphasizing the benefits of healthy eating, regular exercise, and overall well-being instead of solely focusing on weight or appearance is empowering.

Media Literacy and Realistic Standards: Educating oneself about media manipulation and promoting realistic body standards can counter the negative impact of societal pressures on body image. Embracing diverse representations of beauty helps in accepting various body types.

Conclusion

Exploring the psychological aspects of weight management involves understanding and addressing emotional eating patterns, overcoming mental barriers, and cultivating a positive body image. Emotional eating often serves as a coping mechanism, necessitating awareness and alternative strategies for managing emotions. Mental barriers can hinder progress, requiring a shift in mindset and seeking support. Fostering a positive body image involves promoting self-acceptance, emphasizing health over appearance, and being critical of unrealistic societal standards. By addressing these psychological factors, individuals can foster a healthier relationship with food, exercise, and their bodies, promoting holistic well-being.

Understanding Macro and Micro-Nutrients in Nutrition

Importance of Macronutrients

Macronutrients Defined: Macronutrients are essential nutrients required by the body in relatively large quantities to sustain energy production and support bodily functions. They include carbohydrates, proteins, and fats.

Carbohydrates: Carbs serve as the body's primary source of energy. They're found in various foods like grains, fruits, vegetables, and dairy products. Different forms of carbohydrates exist, including simple sugars, complex starches, and dietary fiber.

Proteins: Proteins are fundamental for building and repairing tissues, producing enzymes and hormones, and supporting immune function. Foods rich in protein include meat, fish, eggs, dairy, legumes, nuts, and seeds.

Fats: Dietary fats are vital for energy, absorbing fat-soluble vitamins, insulating organs, and maintaining cell structure. Healthy fats can be found in sources such as avocados, nuts, seeds, olive oil, and fatty fish.

Role of Micronutrients

Micronutrients Defined: Micronutrients are essential vitamins and minerals required by the body in smaller quantities for various physiological functions, including metabolism, immune support, and overall health. They include vitamins (A, B, C, D, E, K) and minerals (calcium, iron, magnesium, zinc, etc.).

Vitamins: Vitamins are organic compounds essential for growth, development, and various metabolic processes. They serve as antioxidants, aid in energy production, and support the immune system. Sources of vitamins include fruits, vegetables, dairy, and fortified foods.

Minerals: Minerals are inorganic elements critical for bone health, nerve function, muscle contraction, and fluid balance. They're obtained from a variety of foods such as leafy greens, nuts, seeds, dairy products, and seafood.

Understanding Macronutrient Functionality

Carbohydrates: Energy Source and Beyond

Energy Source: Carbohydrates are the body's primary fuel, providing readily available energy for physical activities and brain function.

Fiber: Dietary fiber, a type of carbohydrate, aids digestion, promotes satiety, regulates blood sugar levels, and supports heart health. It's found in fruits, vegetables, whole grains, and legumes.

Proteins: Building Blocks of Life

Tissue Repair and Growth: Proteins are composed of amino acids, which are vital for building and repairing tissues, supporting muscle growth, and maintaining overall body structure.

Enzymes and Hormones: Proteins serve as enzymes that facilitate biochemical reactions and as hormones that regulate various bodily functions.

Fats: Essential for Health

Energy Reserve: Fats serve as a concentrated energy source, providing insulation and protecting vital organs. Healthy fats like omega-3 fatty acids support heart health and brain function.

Absorption of Nutrients: Fat-soluble vitamins (A, D, E, K) require dietary fats for absorption and utilization within the body.

Role and Function of Micronutrients

Vitamins: Multifaceted Health Support

Vitamin A: Essential for vision, immune function, and skin health. Found in carrots, sweet potatoes, and leafy greens.

Vitamin C: Acts as an antioxidant, supports immune health, and aids in collagen formation. Abundant in citrus fruits, berries, and bell peppers.

Vitamin D: Vital for bone health, immune function, and calcium absorption. Sunlight exposure and fortified dairy products are primary sources.

Minerals: Vital for Various Functions

Calcium: Critical for bone health, muscle function, and nerve transmission. Found in dairy products, leafy greens, and fortified foods.

Iron: Essential for oxygen transport in the blood and energy production. Sources include red meat, beans, and leafy greens.

Zinc: Supports immune function, wound healing, and protein synthesis. Available in meat, shellfish, nuts, and seeds.

Balancing Macro and Micro-Nutrients for Optimal Health

Importance of a Balanced Diet

Balanced Nutrition: Consuming a variety of foods rich in macronutrients and micronutrients ensures adequate intake for optimal health and well-being.

Portion Control: Maintaining portion sizes and understanding nutritional needs based on individual requirements helps in achieving a balanced diet.

Diverse Food Choices: Incorporating a wide array of fruits, vegetables, whole grains, lean proteins, healthy fats, and dairy or dairy alternatives helps in obtaining essential nutrients.

Conclusion

Understanding the roles of macronutrients and micronutrients in nutrition is crucial for maintaining optimal health. Macronutrients such as carbohydrates, proteins, and fats provide energy and serve essential structural functions, while micronutrients, including vitamins and minerals, are vital for various physiological processes and overall well-being. A balanced diet rich in diverse nutrients is key to supporting bodily functions, promoting health, and preventing deficiencies.

Importance of Macronutrients in Weight Control

Role of Carbohydrates

Energy Source: Carbohydrates serve as the primary energy source for the body. Their role in providing readily available energy is crucial for fueling daily activities and workouts, supporting weight control by managing energy intake.

Choosing the Right Carbs: Opting for complex carbohydrates found in whole grains, fruits, vegetables, and legumes provides sustained energy release, prevents blood sugar spikes, and helps in maintaining satiety.

Impact of Proteins

Muscle Maintenance and Satiation: Proteins play a vital role in muscle repair, growth, and maintenance. Higher protein intake aids in preserving lean muscle mass during weight loss, promotes satiety, and supports metabolic function.

Balancing Protein Sources: Including lean proteins from sources like poultry, fish, tofu, legumes, and dairy in meals helps control appetite and supports weight management efforts.

Contribution of Fats

Satiety and Nutrient Absorption: Dietary fats contribute to satiety, help in the absorption of fat-soluble vitamins, and provide a sense of fullness, reducing overall calorie intake.

Healthy Fats for Weight Control: Incorporating healthy fats like those found in avocados, nuts, seeds, olive oil, and fatty fish aids in weight management by promoting satiety and supporting overall health.

Role of Micronutrients in Metabolism

Vitamins and Metabolism

B Vitamins: B-complex vitamins (B1, B2, B3, B6, B12) play a vital role in converting food into energy and supporting metabolic processes. They facilitate the breakdown of macronutrients, aiding in energy production.

Vitamin D: Vitamin D deficiency may impact metabolism and lead to weight gain. Adequate levels of vitamin D are crucial for regulating metabolism and supporting weight control.

Minerals and Metabolic Function

Calcium: Calcium is involved in regulating metabolic processes related to fat metabolism. Consuming adequate calcium supports weight management efforts.

Iron: Iron plays a role in the transportation of oxygen to cells, aiding in energy production and supporting metabolic functions.

Creating Balanced Meals for Weight Management

Building a Balanced Plate

Incorporating Macronutrients: Crafting meals that contain a balance of carbohydrates, proteins, and healthy fats is key to promoting satiety, regulating blood sugar levels, and controlling cravings.

Portion Control: Being mindful of portion sizes ensures balanced macronutrient intake without excessive calorie consumption, supporting weight control goals.

Emphasizing Micronutrient-Rich Foods

Diverse Food Choices: Including a variety of fruits, vegetables, whole grains, lean proteins, and healthy fats in meals ensures a rich supply of micronutrients essential for metabolic functions and overall health.

Meal Planning for Nutrient Variety: Planning meals that encompass different food groups allows for a broad spectrum of vitamins and minerals, aiding in overall metabolic health.

Conclusion

Understanding the importance of macronutrients, including carbohydrates, proteins, and fats, in weight control is crucial for structuring balanced meals that support energy needs and satiety. Additionally, recognizing the role of micronutrients, such as vitamins and minerals, in metabolism highlights their significance in supporting metabolic functions vital for weight management. Creating balanced meals that combine macronutrients in appropriate proportions while emphasizing micronutrient-rich foods facilitates healthy eating patterns conducive to weight control.

UNDERSTANDING WEIGHT MANAGEMENT: 2024 EDITION

CHAPTER 3

Innovative Diets: A Paradigm Shift in Weight Control

1. Plant-Based Diets

Principles: Plant-based diets focus on consuming predominantly or exclusively plant-derived foods, including fruits, vegetables, whole grains, nuts, seeds, and legumes. They emphasize the health benefits of plant foods while often minimizing or excluding animal products.

Benefits for Weight Control: Plant-based diets are rich in fiber, vitamins, and antioxidants while typically lower in saturated fats and cholesterol. Studies suggest they may contribute to weight management by promoting satiety, reducing calorie intake, and supporting a healthy metabolism.

2. Intermittent Fasting

Approach: Intermittent fasting involves cycling between periods of eating and fasting. Common methods include the 16/8 method (eating within an 8-hour window), alternate-day fasting, or periodic fasting (such as the 5:2 diet, consuming a limited number of calories on specific days).

Weight Management Benefits: Intermittent fasting may aid weight control by regulating insulin sensitivity, promoting fat oxidation, and supporting metabolic health. Some individuals find it helpful in reducing overall calorie intake without strict dietary restrictions.

3. Mediterranean Diet

Foundation: The Mediterranean diet is inspired by traditional eating patterns in countries bordering the Mediterranean Sea. It emphasizes plant-based foods, healthy fats (such as olive oil), moderate consumption of fish, poultry, dairy, and occasional red wine.

Weight Control Advantages: Known for its heart-healthy benefits, the Mediterranean diet may aid in weight management due to its emphasis on whole foods, healthy fats, and a balance of nutrients. It promotes satiety and supports overall health.

4. Ketogenic Diet

Principles: The ketogenic diet is a low-carbohydrate, high-fat diet that aims to induce a metabolic state called ketosis, where the body utilizes ketones (derived from fat) as its primary energy source. It involves drastically reducing carbohydrate intake and increasing fats.

Weight Control Mechanism: By limiting carbohydrates, the ketogenic diet prompts the body to burn fat for energy, potentially leading to weight loss. However, its restrictive nature might pose challenges in adhering to the diet long-term.

5. DASH Diet

Approach: DASH (Dietary Approaches to Stop Hypertension) emphasizes consuming foods rich in nutrients like potassium, calcium, protein, and fiber while limiting sodium intake. It emphasizes fruits, vegetables, whole grains, and lean proteins.

Weight Management Benefits: The DASH diet, known for its heart-healthy benefits, supports weight management by promoting nutrient-dense foods, reducing sodium-induced water retention, and improving overall dietary quality.

6. Flexitarian Diet

Foundation: A flexible approach combining the words "flexible" and "vegetarian," the flexitarian diet encourages plant-based eating while allowing occasional consumption of meat and other animal products.

Weight Control Aspects: Flexitarianism promotes the health benefits of plant-based foods while providing flexibility, making it easier for individuals to adopt and sustain healthier eating patterns conducive to weight control.

Innovation and Personalization in Diet Choices

Individualization of Diets

Personalized Nutrition: Tailoring diets to individual preferences, lifestyle, health conditions, and cultural factors is crucial. This approach acknowledges that not all diets suit everyone and allows for adaptations that align with personal needs and goals.

Innovation in Food Technology: Advancements in food technology have introduced innovative plant-based substitutes, such as meat alternatives made from plant proteins, contributing to more diverse and sustainable dietary options for weight control.

Behavior Modification and Long-Term Adherence

Focus on Behavioral Change: Innovative diets often emphasize behavioral modifications, encouraging a shift in mindset and lifestyle habits rather than solely focusing on restrictive eating patterns.

Sustainability and Longevity: A key aspect of innovative diets for weight control is their sustainability. Diets that individuals can adopt and maintain long-term, without feeling overly restricted, tend to yield more sustainable weight management outcomes.

Conclusion

Innovative diets for weight control encompass a diverse range of approaches, each emphasizing unique principles and potential benefits. Whether it's plant-based diets, intermittent fasting, Mediterranean or ketogenic diets, the key lies in understanding individual needs, preferences, and the ability to maintain these dietary patterns in the long run. By embracing innovation, personalized nutrition, behavioral modifications, and sustainable approaches, individuals can explore and adopt diets that suit their lifestyle, preferences, and health goals for effective and sustainable weight management.

Exploring Emerging Diets

Intermittent Fasting: Revamping Eating Patterns

Approach: Intermittent fasting involves cycling between periods of eating and fasting. The most common methods include the 16/8 method (eating within an 8-hour window) and alternate-day fasting.

Benefits: Intermittent fasting may promote weight loss by regulating insulin sensitivity, boosting fat burning, and controlling calorie intake. It also shows potential in supporting metabolic health and reducing inflammation.

Embracing Plant-Based Diets

Principles: Plant-based diets center around consuming predominantly plant-derived foods while minimizing or excluding animal products. They emphasize whole grains, fruits, vegetables, nuts, seeds, and legumes.

Weight Management: Plant-based diets are rich in fiber, antioxidants, and nutrients while typically lower in saturated fats. Studies suggest they may aid in weight control by enhancing satiety and supporting overall health.

Understanding the Ketogenic Diet and Weight Effects

Ketogenic Diet: A Low-Carb Approach

Principles: The ketogenic diet involves drastically reducing carbohydrate intake and increasing fats to induce ketosis, a metabolic state where the body primarily uses ketones for energy.

Weight Effects: Ketogenic diets may promote weight loss by shifting the body's primary fuel source to fats, thereby encouraging fat burning for energy. However, long-term adherence and potential side effects need consideration.

Ketogenic Diet and Metabolic Changes

Metabolic Shift: By limiting carbohydrates, the body switches from using glucose for energy to utilizing stored fat as its primary fuel source, potentially leading to weight loss.

Appetite Regulation: Ketosis may affect appetite regulation and satiety hormones, which could contribute to reduced hunger and calorie intake, aiding weight management efforts.

Customized Diet Plans for Different Lifestyles

Adapting Diets to Lifestyles

Busy Lifestyles: For individuals with hectic schedules, meal prepping and planning help maintain dietary consistency. Opting for grab-and-go healthy snacks and easy-to-prepare meals supports adherence to a chosen diet.

Athletic and Active Lifestyles: Customized diets for athletes may focus on optimizing nutrient intake to fuel workouts, support muscle recovery, and maintain energy levels. Tailoring macronutrients to performance goals is crucial.

Dietary Plans for Health Conditions

Medical Considerations: Customized diets are essential for individuals with specific health conditions like diabetes, cardiovascular issues, or food allergies. Tailoring dietary plans to accommodate these conditions is vital for overall health and well-being.

Cultural and Ethical Considerations: Customized diets also consider cultural preferences and ethical choices. Flexibility in diet plans accommodates diverse cultural practices and personal beliefs surrounding food choices.

Conclusion

Exploring emerging diets like intermittent fasting and plant-based diets reveals diverse approaches to weight management, each with distinct principles and potential benefits. The ketogenic diet, with its low-carbohydrate, high-fat approach, demonstrates potential effects on weight through metabolic changes. Customized diet plans tailored to various lifestyles, health conditions, and personal preferences ensure dietary adherence and support overall well-being. Embracing these emerging diets requires a nuanced understanding of their mechanisms, potential effects, and the importance of personalized approaches to suit individual needs.

Exploring the Relationship Between Gut Health and Weight Management

Understanding Gut Health

Gut Microbiota: The gut harbors trillions of microbes collectively known as the gut microbiota, consisting of bacteria, fungi, viruses, and other microorganisms. This complex ecosystem plays a pivotal role in various bodily functions.

Microbiome Diversity: A diverse and balanced gut microbiome contributes to overall health, aiding in digestion, nutrient absorption, immune function, and even influencing mental health.

Gut Microbiota and Weight Regulation

Role in Metabolism: Emerging research suggests that the gut microbiota influences metabolism and energy regulation, impacting how the body stores fat, extracts energy from food, and regulates appetite.

Impact on Inflammation and Hormones: Imbalances in the gut microbiota can lead to inflammation and affect hormone levels related to appetite control, potentially contributing to weight gain or difficulties in weight management.

Factors Influencing Gut Health and Weight

Diet and Gut Microbiota

Dietary Influence: The composition of the gut microbiota is strongly influenced by dietary choices. Diets rich in fiber, diverse fruits, vegetables, and fermented foods support a more diverse and beneficial gut microbiome.

Effects of Macronutrients: Different macronutrients impact gut health differently. For instance, fiber promotes the growth of beneficial bacteria, while excessive intake of sugar or processed foods may negatively affect gut microbial diversity.

Lifestyle and Gut Health

Physical Activity: Regular exercise positively influences gut health, promoting microbial diversity and reducing inflammation, which may indirectly impact weight management.

Stress Management: Chronic stress can alter the gut microbiota, potentially affecting weight regulation. Techniques like meditation, yoga, or mindfulness may support gut health and aid in weight control.

Gut Health Interventions for Weight Management

Probiotics and Prebiotics

Probiotics: These are live beneficial bacteria found in certain foods or supplements. They support gut health by introducing beneficial microbes, potentially aiding digestion and immune function.

Prebiotics: Prebiotics are dietary fibers that serve as fuel for beneficial gut bacteria. Foods like garlic, onions, bananas, and whole grains contain prebiotic fibers that support a healthy gut environment.

Dietary Modifications for Gut Health

Fiber-Rich Foods: Incorporating high-fiber foods like whole grains, fruits, vegetables, legumes, and nuts promotes gut health by nourishing beneficial gut bacteria and aiding digestion.

Fermented Foods: Including fermented foods like yogurt, kefir, kimchi, sauerkraut, and kombucha introduces probiotics that support gut microbial diversity.

Personalized Approaches for Gut Health and Weight

Individualized Gut Health Assessments

Microbiome Testing: Advanced technologies allow for analyzing an individual's gut microbiome composition, offering insights into specific microbial imbalances or deficiencies.

Tailored Dietary Plans: Understanding an individual's unique gut composition enables the formulation of personalized dietary recommendations to support gut health and weight management goals.

Long-Term Lifestyle Modifications

Sustainable Changes: Incorporating long-term lifestyle changes that prioritize a balanced diet, regular physical activity, stress reduction, and adequate sleep supports a healthy gut environment and sustainable weight management.

Gradual Adaptations: Gradually introducing dietary changes and lifestyle modifications allows the gut microbiota to adapt and thrive, supporting a lasting impact on gut health and weight regulation.

Conclusion

The intricate relationship between gut health and weight management underscores the importance of nurturing a balanced and diverse gut microbiome. The gut microbiota influences various aspects of metabolism, inflammation, and hormonal regulation, which in turn can impact weight regulation and overall health. Implementing interventions such as probiotics, prebiotics, dietary modifications, and personalized approaches tailored to individual gut health supports a healthy gut environment and aids in weight management. Embracing sustainable lifestyle modifications that prioritize gut health lays the foundation for achieving and maintaining a healthy weight and overall well-being.

Understanding and nurturing gut health is integral to effective weight management. Implementing strategies to support a diverse gut microbiome through dietary choices, lifestyle modifications, and personalized interventions not only aids in weight control but also contributes to overall health and well-being.

The Interplay Between Gut Microbiota and Weight

Impact of Gut Microbiota Composition

Microbial Diversity: A diverse gut microbiota contributes to overall health, influencing metabolism, energy regulation, and nutrient absorption. Imbalances in microbial composition may be associated with weight-related issues.

Influence on Metabolic Processes: The gut microbiota plays a crucial role in metabolizing nutrients, producing short-chain fatty acids (SCFAs), regulating inflammation, and impacting appetite control, all of which can influence weight management.

Probiotics, Prebiotics, and Their Impact on Weight Regulation

Probiotics: Beneficial Bacteria for Gut Health

Role in Gut Health: Probiotics are live beneficial bacteria that, when consumed in adequate amounts, promote a healthy gut environment by bolstering the balance of beneficial microbes.

Weight Management Potential: Some studies suggest that certain probiotic strains may aid in weight regulation by influencing appetite control, reducing inflammation, and modulating energy metabolism.

Prebiotics: Fuel for Gut Microbes

Supporting Gut Microbiota: Prebiotics are non-digestible fibers that act as food for beneficial gut bacteria, supporting their growth and activity.

Weight Control Effects: Prebiotics, found in foods like chicory root, garlic, onions, and bananas, can promote a healthier gut environment, potentially impacting weight by enhancing satiety and aiding in the absorption of nutrients.

Strategies to Improve Gut Health for Weight Control

Dietary Modifications for Gut Health

Fiber-Rich Foods: Including a variety of high-fiber foods such as fruits, vegetables, whole grains, legumes, and nuts supports gut health by nourishing beneficial gut bacteria.

Fermented Foods: Incorporating fermented foods like yogurt, kefir, sauerkraut, kimchi, and kombucha introduces probiotics that support a diverse gut microbiome.

Probiotic and Prebiotic Supplementation

Supplement Considerations: Probiotic supplements containing specific strains (such as Lactobacillus and Bifidobacterium) and prebiotic supplements may help improve gut health, but individual responses can vary.

Consultation and Dosage: Consulting with a healthcare professional or a registered dietitian can help determine suitable probiotic or prebiotic supplementation and dosage for individual needs.

Lifestyle Factors Impacting Gut Health

Balanced Diet: Consuming a diverse range of nutrients through a balanced diet supports gut microbial diversity, promoting a healthier gut environment.

Physical Activity: Regular exercise positively influences gut health by enhancing microbial diversity and reducing inflammation, indirectly impacting weight management.

Conclusion

The intricate relationship between gut microbiota and weight underscores the importance of fostering a diverse and balanced gut environment for effective weight control. Probiotics and prebiotics play pivotal roles in supporting gut health, potentially influencing weight regulation through mechanisms such as appetite control, inflammation modulation, and metabolic processes. Strategies focusing on dietary modifications, incorporating probiotics and prebiotics, and considering lifestyle factors promote a healthier gut microbiome, offering promising avenues for weight management. However, individual responses to these strategies may vary, emphasizing the importance of personalized approaches to improve gut health and support weight control.

Understanding the intricate interplay between gut microbiota and weight provides insights into strategies for effective weight management. Embracing dietary modifications, incorporating probiotics and prebiotics, and considering lifestyle factors that support a healthy gut environment contribute to fostering optimal gut health and may aid in weight regulation. Customized approaches tailored to individual needs pave the way for improved gut health, thereby supporting overall well-being and sustainable weight control.

The Importance of Exercise and Physical Activity

Physical Activity for Overall Health

Enhanced Physical Fitness: Regular physical activity improves cardiovascular endurance, muscular strength, flexibility, and overall physical fitness levels.

Disease Prevention: Engaging in regular exercise lowers the risk of chronic diseases such as heart disease, diabetes, hypertension, obesity, and certain cancers.

Mental Health and Well-being

Mood Enhancement: Physical activity stimulates the production of endorphins, promoting feelings of happiness and reducing stress, anxiety, and symptoms of depression.

Cognitive Function: Exercise supports cognitive function, memory, and brain health, potentially reducing the risk of cognitive decline with age.

Understanding Different Types of Exercise

Aerobic Exercise

Cardiovascular Benefits: Activities like brisk walking, running, cycling, swimming, and dancing elevate heart rate, improving cardiovascular health and endurance.

Weight Management: Aerobic exercises burn calories, aiding in weight management by promoting fat loss and supporting a healthy metabolism.

Strength Training

Muscle Development: Weightlifting, resistance band exercises, and bodyweight exercises strengthen muscles, enhance bone density, and improve overall strength.

Metabolic Impact: Strength training boosts metabolism, facilitating fat loss, and supports the maintenance of lean muscle mass.

Flexibility and Balance

Improved Range of Motion: Stretching, yoga, and tai chi improve flexibility, joint mobility, and muscle elasticity, reducing the risk of injuries.

Enhanced Stability: Activities focusing on balance, such as specific yoga poses or balance exercises, contribute to improved stability and fall prevention, especially in older adults.

Benefits of Regular Exercise

Weight Management and Metabolism

Caloric Expenditure: Regular physical activity burns calories, supporting weight management by contributing to a calorie deficit when combined with a balanced diet.

Metabolic Rate: Exercise increases metabolism, allowing for more efficient calorie burning even at rest, aiding in weight control efforts.

Heart Health and Disease Prevention

Cardiovascular Benefits: Regular exercise strengthens the heart muscle, improves blood circulation, and reduces the risk of heart disease and stroke.

Blood Pressure Control: Physical activity helps in lowering blood pressure, contributing to overall cardiovascular health.

Incorporating Physical Activity into Daily Life

Establishing a Routine

Consistency: Creating a regular exercise routine enhances adherence, making physical activity a habitual part of daily life.

Variety: Incorporating diverse exercises maintains interest, prevents boredom, and targets different muscle groups, enhancing overall fitness.

Finding Enjoyment in Exercise

Choose Activities Wisely: Engage in activities that align with personal interests, making exercise enjoyable and sustainable.

Group Activities: Participating in group fitness classes, sports, or activities with friends fosters motivation and social interaction.

Conclusion

Exercise and physical activity are integral components of a healthy lifestyle, offering a myriad of physical, mental, and emotional benefits. Engaging in regular exercise, encompassing aerobic, strength, flexibility, and balance training, supports overall health by enhancing physical fitness, aiding in weight management, reducing the risk of chronic diseases, and promoting mental well-being. Incorporating physical activity into daily life through a consistent routine, variety in exercises, and finding enjoyment in activities ensures sustained adherence, contributing to lifelong health and vitality.

Exercise and physical activity form the cornerstone of a healthy lifestyle, offering multifaceted benefits for overall well-being. Embracing regular exercise in various forms supports physical fitness, weight management, disease prevention, mental health, and overall quality of life. Making exercise a consistent and enjoyable part of daily routines fosters a lifelong commitment to health and vitality.

The Importance of Exercise and Physical Activity

Physical Activity for Overall Health

Enhanced Physical Fitness: Regular physical activity improves cardiovascular endurance, muscular strength, flexibility, and overall physical fitness levels.

Disease Prevention: Engaging in regular exercise lowers the risk of chronic diseases such as heart disease, diabetes, hypertension, obesity, and certain cancers.

Mental Health and Well-being

Mood Enhancement: Physical activity stimulates the production of endorphins, promoting feelings of happiness and reducing stress, anxiety, and symptoms of depression.

Cognitive Function: Exercise supports cognitive function, memory, and brain health, potentially reducing the risk of cognitive decline with age.

Understanding Different Types of Exercise

Aerobic Exercise

Cardiovascular Benefits: Activities like brisk walking, running, cycling, swimming, and dancing elevate heart rate, improving cardiovascular health and endurance.

Weight Management: Aerobic exercises burn calories, aiding in weight management by promoting fat loss and supporting a healthy metabolism.

Strength Training

Muscle Development: Weightlifting, resistance band exercises, and bodyweight exercises strengthen muscles, enhance bone density, and improve overall strength.

Metabolic Impact: Strength training boosts metabolism, facilitating fat loss, and supports the maintenance of lean muscle mass.

Flexibility and Balance

Improved Range of Motion: Stretching, yoga, and tai chi improve flexibility, joint mobility, and muscle elasticity, reducing the risk of injuries.

Enhanced Stability: Activities focusing on balance, such as specific yoga poses or balance exercises, contribute to improved stability and fall prevention, especially in older adults.

Benefits of Regular Exercise

Weight Management and Metabolism

Caloric Expenditure: Regular physical activity burns calories, supporting weight management by contributing to a calorie deficit when combined with a balanced diet.

Metabolic Rate: Exercise increases metabolism, allowing for more efficient calorie burning even at rest, aiding in weight control efforts.

Heart Health and Disease Prevention

Cardiovascular Benefits: Regular exercise strengthens the heart muscle, improves blood circulation, and reduces the risk of heart disease and stroke.

Blood Pressure Control: Physical activity helps in lowering blood pressure, contributing to overall cardiovascular health.

Incorporating Physical Activity into Daily Life

Establishing a Routine

Consistency: Creating a regular exercise routine enhances adherence, making physical activity a habitual part of daily life.

Variety: Incorporating diverse exercises maintains interest, prevents boredom, and targets different muscle groups, enhancing overall fitness.

Finding Enjoyment in Exercise

Choose Activities Wisely: Engage in activities that align with personal interests, making exercise enjoyable and sustainable.

Group Activities: Participating in group fitness classes, sports, or activities with friends fosters motivation and social interaction.

Conclusion

Exercise and physical activity are integral components of a healthy lifestyle, offering a myriad of physical, mental, and emotional benefits. Engaging in regular exercise, encompassing aerobic, strength, flexibility, and balance training, supports overall health by enhancing physical fitness, aiding in weight management, reducing the risk of chronic diseases, and promoting mental well-being. Incorporating physical activity into daily life through a consistent routine, variety in exercises, and finding enjoyment in activities ensures sustained adherence, contributing to lifelong health and vitality.

Exercise and physical activity form the cornerstone of a healthy lifestyle, offering multifaceted benefits for overall well-being. Embracing regular exercise in various forms supports physical fitness, weight management, disease prevention, mental health, and overall quality of life. Making exercise a consistent and enjoyable part of daily routines fosters a lifelong commitment to health and vitality.

UNDERSTANDING WEIGHT MANAGEMENT: 2024 EDITION

CHAPTER 4

Impact of Different Exercise Types on Weight Management

Aerobic Exercise for Weight Loss

Caloric Expenditure: Activities like running, cycling, or swimming facilitate calorie burning, aiding weight management by creating a caloric deficit when combined with a balanced diet.

Fat Burning: Aerobic exercises primarily rely on fat as a fuel source, making them effective for fat loss and supporting overall weight management goals.

Strength Training and Weight Control

Metabolic Impact: Resistance training, by building lean muscle mass, boosts metabolism, promoting ongoing calorie burn even at rest, contributing to weight management.

Body Composition Changes: While not directly reducing weight, resistance training supports fat loss and enhances muscle definition, improving body composition.

High-Intensity Interval Training (HIIT) and Its Effectiveness

HIIT for Weight Loss

Short, Intense Bursts: HIIT involves short bursts of intense exercise followed by brief recovery periods, effectively elevating heart rate and calorie burn in a shorter time.

Metabolic Rate Increase: HIIT sessions elevate post-exercise oxygen consumption (EPOC), causing a sustained increase in metabolism, facilitating calorie burn even after the workout.

Efficiency and Fat Loss

Effective Fat Burning: HIIT workouts target stubborn fat areas, aiding in fat loss and supporting weight management while preserving muscle mass.

Time-Efficient: HIIT workouts, typically shorter in duration but intense, offer a time-efficient approach to burning calories and improving cardiovascular fitness.

Integrating Resistance Training for Weight Loss

Muscle Development and Metabolism

Muscle Mass Impact: Resistance training promotes muscle growth, which, in turn, boosts metabolism and aids in long-term weight control by facilitating ongoing calorie burn.

Improved Body Composition: Building lean muscle through resistance training contributes to improved body composition, enhancing aesthetics and overall health.

Effective Caloric Expenditure

Calorie Burning Potential: While resistance training doesn't burn as many calories during the workout as aerobic exercises, it contributes to increased calorie expenditure during and after exercise due to muscle repair and growth.

Combination Benefits: Combining resistance training with aerobic exercises creates a holistic approach to weight management, optimizing fat loss, and muscle gain.

Combining Exercise Types for Weight Management

Holistic Approach to Weight Loss

Synergistic Effects: Integrating both aerobic exercises and resistance training provides comprehensive benefits, optimizing fat loss, preserving muscle mass, and enhancing overall fitness.

Varied Workouts: Alternating between different exercise types prevents plateaus, challenges the body, and ensures overall physical fitness improvement.

Tailoring Exercise Regimens

Individual Preferences: Customizing workouts based on personal preferences ensures adherence, making exercise enjoyable and sustainable.

Progressive Overload: Gradually increasing the intensity and complexity of workouts aids in continuous improvements in strength, endurance, and overall fitness.

Conclusion

Different types of exercise offer unique benefits for weight management. Aerobic exercises aid in fat burning and calorie expenditure, while resistance training supports muscle development, metabolism, and improved body composition. High-Intensity Interval Training (HIIT) provides an efficient way to burn calories and improve cardiovascular fitness. Integrating these exercise modalities into a holistic approach supports comprehensive weight management, ensuring fat loss, muscle preservation, and overall fitness enhancement. Customizing exercise regimens based on individual preferences and gradually progressing workouts fosters sustained adherence and long-term success in weight control efforts.

Different types of exercises, from aerobic to resistance training and HIIT, offer distinct advantages for weight management. Incorporating a balanced mix of these exercises into a tailored fitness regimen contributes to holistic weight control, facilitating fat loss, preserving muscle mass, and improving overall physical fitness. Customizing workouts and progressing gradually ensures sustained adherence, making exercise a fundamental component of successful weight management strategies.

Non-Traditional Approaches to Fitness

1. Bodyweight Training

Principle: Bodyweight exercises utilize one's body weight for resistance, requiring minimal or no equipment. These exercises, like push-ups, squats, and planks, improve strength and flexibility.

Benefits: Bodyweight training is convenient, cost-effective, and adaptable to various fitness levels, making it accessible for individuals with limited space or equipment.

2. Animal Flow Workouts

Approach: Inspired by animal movements, this workout involves fluid, ground-based movements like bear crawls, crab walks, and ape reaches to enhance strength, flexibility, and body control.

Benefits: Animal flow workouts improve mobility, coordination, and stability while providing a fun and unconventional way to exercise.

3. Parkour and Free Running

Principle: Parkour involves moving through urban environments by navigating obstacles creatively, while free running focuses on acrobatic movements, flips, and jumps within the same context.

Benefits: These activities improve agility, strength, and spatial awareness, emphasizing adaptability and creativity in movement.

4. Trampoline Workouts

Approach: Trampoline workouts involve exercises performed on mini-trampolines, offering a low-impact cardio workout that includes bouncing, jumping, and balance exercises.

Benefits: Trampoline workouts are gentle on joints, enhance cardiovascular health, and improve balance and coordination while being enjoyable and engaging.

5. Pole Fitness

Approach: Pole fitness combines dance, acrobatics, and strength training using a vertical pole. It involves spins, climbs, and inversions, targeting upper body and core strength.

Benefits: Pole fitness improves strength, flexibility, and body awareness, promoting confidence and gracefulness while challenging individuals both physically and mentally.

Non-Conventional Fitness Trends

1. Virtual Fitness Classes

Concept: Virtual fitness classes provide online access to workouts led by instructors, allowing individuals to exercise at home or on-the-go using streaming services or apps.

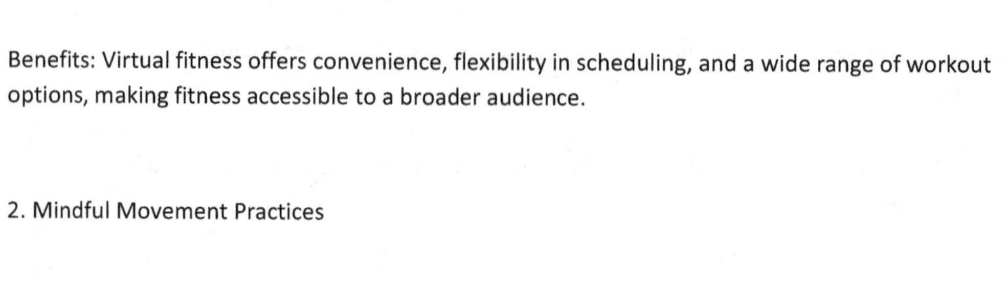

Benefits: Virtual fitness offers convenience, flexibility in scheduling, and a wide range of workout options, making fitness accessible to a broader audience.

2. Mindful Movement Practices

Incorporation: Mindful movement practices such as yoga, Pilates, and tai chi emphasize breathwork, body awareness, and mental focus alongside physical exercises.

Benefits: These practices enhance flexibility, balance, and mental well-being, promoting stress reduction and relaxation.

Exploring Unconventional Fitness Modalities

1. Aquatic Workouts

Water-Based Exercise: Aquatic workouts involve movements in water, like swimming, water aerobics, or aqua cycling, providing resistance and low-impact cardio.

Benefits: These workouts are joint-friendly, improve cardiovascular fitness, and offer resistance training without excess strain on the body.

2. Electrical Muscle Stimulation (EMS) Training

Technology Integration: EMS involves using electrical impulses to stimulate muscle contractions while performing exercises, intensifying workouts and targeting specific muscle groups.

Benefits: EMS training may improve muscle strength, aid in rehabilitation, and optimize time efficiency by providing an intense workout in a shorter duration.

Conclusion

Non-traditional approaches to fitness encompass a diverse range of unconventional workouts, alternative fitness trends, and unique exercise modalities. These innovative methods offer distinct benefits, from enhancing strength, flexibility, and cardiovascular fitness to promoting mental well-being and offering convenience and accessibility. Embracing non-traditional fitness modalities introduces variety, challenges the body in new ways, and fosters enjoyment and engagement in exercise routines. As individuals seek diverse and personalized fitness experiences, these non-conventional approaches continue to expand horizons, providing novel ways to achieve overall health and wellness.

Non-traditional approaches to fitness offer a diverse array of innovative workouts and alternative fitness trends that cater to various interests, abilities, and preferences. Exploring these unconventional methods introduces excitement, variety, and effectiveness to fitness routines, fostering engagement and supporting overall health and well-being. Incorporating these non-conventional modalities into fitness regimens encourages diversity, challenges the body in unique ways, and enhances the overall fitness experience.

Mind-Body Exercises for Weight Management

1. Yoga for Weight Control

Principles: Yoga combines physical postures, breathwork, and meditation, promoting relaxation, flexibility, and mindfulness.

Weight Management Benefits: Certain yoga styles (e.g., Vinyasa, Power Yoga) provide moderate aerobic exercise, promoting calorie burn and stress reduction, which may aid weight control by managing cortisol levels.

2. Pilates and Weight Loss

Approach: Pilates focuses on core strength, stability, and controlled movements, enhancing muscular endurance and flexibility.

Weight Management Benefits: Pilates can improve muscle tone and overall body composition, supporting weight management indirectly by increasing muscle mass and metabolic rate.

Integrating Technology into Fitness Routines

1. Fitness Apps and Wearable Devices

Functionality: Fitness apps and wearable devices track physical activity, heart rate, calories burned, and offer guided workouts, enhancing accountability and motivation.

Weight Management Support: These tools provide data insights, goal setting, and personalized workouts, aiding individuals in maintaining a consistent exercise routine for weight control.

2. Virtual Fitness Platforms

Online Workouts: Virtual fitness platforms offer live or pre-recorded classes, ranging from HIIT to yoga, enabling individuals to access diverse workouts from home.

Convenience and Engagement: These platforms provide convenience, flexibility in scheduling, and diverse workout options, enhancing engagement and adherence to fitness routines.

Outdoor Activities and Their Role in Weight Control

1. Hiking and Weight Management

Physical Benefits: Hiking engages various muscle groups, offers cardiovascular exercise, and burns calories, contributing to weight management.

Mental Well-being: Being outdoors improves mental health, reduces stress, and boosts mood, indirectly supporting healthy habits conducive to weight control.

2. Cycling for Fitness

Cardiovascular Exercise: Cycling, whether on roads or trails, provides a low-impact cardio workout, burning calories and improving cardiovascular health.

Variety and Enjoyment: Cycling offers variety, can be done alone or in groups, and allows exploration of different terrains, enhancing enjoyment and adherence to exercise routines.

Combining Mind-Body Practices, Technology, and Outdoor Activities

1. Mindful Technology Use

Tech-Assisted Mind-Body Activities: Integrating apps or online platforms offering yoga, meditation, or Pilates classes merges technology with mind-body exercises for holistic well-being.

Outdoor Fitness Apps: Utilizing apps for outdoor activities like hiking or cycling guides individuals in exploring new trails, enhancing the outdoor exercise experience.

2. Mindful Outdoor Workouts

Mindfulness in Nature: Engaging in mind-body exercises outdoors fosters a deeper connection with nature, promoting mental relaxation and stress reduction.

Technology-Assisted Outdoor Fitness: Wearable devices or apps that track outdoor activities provide data insights, encouraging individuals to set and achieve fitness goals effectively.

Conclusion

Mind-body exercises like yoga and Pilates, when combined with technology integration and outdoor activities, offer diverse avenues for weight management. These practices not only contribute to physical fitness but also promote mental well-being, stress reduction, and overall health. Incorporating technology into fitness routines enhances accessibility, motivation, and engagement, while outdoor activities provide opportunities for varied workouts in natural environments. Combining mind-body practices with technology and outdoor exercise offers a holistic approach to weight control, fostering a balance between physical fitness, mental wellness, and enjoyment in fitness pursuits.

Mind-body exercises such as yoga and Pilates, combined with technology integration and outdoor activities, offer multifaceted approaches to weight management. Embracing these practices, whether through mindful movement, tech-assisted workouts, or outdoor fitness activities, supports holistic well-being, promoting physical fitness, mental relaxation, and overall health. The synergy between mind-body exercises, technology, and outdoor activities facilitates a comprehensive approach to weight control, ensuring a balanced and enjoyable fitness journey.

Lifestyle Changes for Sustainable Weight Maintenance

1. Establishing Healthy Dietary Habits

Balanced Nutrition: Focus on a balanced diet comprising whole foods, incorporating ample fruits, vegetables, lean proteins, whole grains, and healthy fats.

Portion Control: Practice mindful eating, pay attention to portion sizes, and listen to hunger and fullness cues to prevent overeating.

2. Maintaining a Regular Exercise Routine

Consistent Physical Activity: Incorporate regular exercise into your routine, aiming for a mix of aerobic, strength training, and flexibility exercises to support overall fitness.

Daily Movement: Engage in non-exercise physical activities, such as taking the stairs, walking, or stretching throughout the day to increase overall daily movement.

3. Behavioral Changes and Mindful Eating

Mindful Eating Practices: Slow down while eating, savoring each bite, and being mindful of hunger and satiety cues to avoid mindless overeating.

Stress Management: Practice stress-reducing techniques like meditation, deep breathing, or yoga to manage stress-related eating behaviors.

4. Setting Realistic Goals and Tracking Progress

Goal Setting: Establish achievable, realistic weight maintenance goals that focus on long-term health rather than rapid weight loss.

Tracking Progress: Monitor weight, measurements, dietary intake, and exercise routines to track progress and make necessary adjustments.

5. Building a Supportive Environment

Social Support: Surround yourself with a supportive network of friends, family, or a community with similar health goals, fostering encouragement and accountability.

Healthy Home Environment: Create a home environment conducive to healthy habits by stocking nutritious foods, planning meals, and promoting physical activity.

6. Prioritizing Sleep and Stress Management

Adequate Sleep: Prioritize quality sleep, aiming for 7-9 hours per night, as inadequate sleep can disrupt appetite-regulating hormones and impact weight management.

Stress Reduction: Manage stress through relaxation techniques, hobbies, or activities that promote mental well-being, reducing the likelihood of stress-related eating.

Sustainable Strategies for Weight Maintenance

1. Gradual Behavior Changes

Slow Adaptations: Implement lifestyle changes gradually, allowing for adjustment and adherence to new habits over time.

Consistency over Perfection: Focus on consistent progress rather than perfection, embracing occasional setbacks as part of the journey.

2. Mindful Eating and Food Choices

Nutrient-Dense Foods: Emphasize whole, nutrient-dense foods, limiting processed and high-calorie, low-nutrient foods to support a balanced diet.

Portion Awareness: Practice portion control, using smaller plates, measuring servings, and being mindful of portion sizes to prevent overconsumption.

3. Regular Physical Activity

Varied Workouts: Engage in a mix of exercises that cater to personal preferences, ensuring enjoyment and adherence to a consistent exercise routine.

Routine Adaptations: Adjust exercise routines periodically to prevent boredom and plateaus, challenging the body and promoting continued progress.

Behavioral Strategies for Long-Term Success

1. Behavioral Modification Techniques

Cognitive Behavioral Therapy (CBT): Consider CBT or counseling to address emotional eating, stress management, and behavioral patterns related to food.

Positive Reinforcement: Celebrate achievements, no matter how small, and reward yourself with non-food-related incentives for reaching milestones.

2. Self-Monitoring and Accountability

Food and Exercise Journaling: Keep a food diary or use apps to track food intake, exercise sessions, and mood, fostering awareness and accountability.

Support Systems: Join support groups, fitness classes, or work with a health coach or nutritionist for guidance, motivation, and accountability.

Conclusion

Sustainable weight maintenance involves adopting healthy lifestyle changes encompassing dietary habits, physical activity, behavioral adjustments, and a supportive environment. Establishing a balanced, nutritious diet, incorporating regular physical activity, practicing mindful eating, setting achievable goals, managing stress, and prioritizing sleep are fundamental aspects. Gradual, consistent changes, coupled with behavioral modification techniques and self-monitoring, foster long-term success in weight maintenance. Embracing a holistic approach to lifestyle changes supports a healthier and more balanced life, ensuring sustained weight management and overall well-being.

Implementing sustainable lifestyle changes, including dietary modifications, regular physical activity, behavioral adjustments, and supportive environments, forms the foundation for successful weight maintenance. By adopting these lifestyle habits and incorporating behavioral strategies, individuals can achieve and sustain weight management goals while promoting overall health and well-being. The key lies in consistency, mindfulness, gradual changes, and a holistic approach to create a sustainable and healthier lifestyle for the long term.

The Impact of Sleep on Weight Management

1. Sleep and Appetite Regulation

Hormonal Regulation: Sleep influences hormones that regulate appetite, such as leptin (suppresses appetite) and ghrelin (stimulates appetite). Inadequate sleep disrupts these hormones, leading to increased hunger and cravings.

Increased Caloric Intake: Sleep deprivation often leads to increased consumption of high-calorie foods and excessive snacking, contributing to weight gain over time.

2. Metabolism and Energy Expenditure

Metabolic Changes: Poor sleep quality or inadequate sleep duration affects metabolism, slowing down the body's ability to process and utilize energy, potentially leading to weight gain.

Reduced Physical Activity: Fatigue from lack of sleep may reduce motivation for physical activity and exercise, further impacting energy expenditure.

3. Insulin Sensitivity and Weight Control

Blood Sugar Regulation: Inadequate sleep affects insulin sensitivity, disrupting blood sugar levels and potentially increasing the risk of insulin resistance and type 2 diabetes.

Impact on Fat Storage: Poor sleep quality may contribute to increased fat storage, particularly around the abdominal area, associated with higher health risks.

The Relationship Between Sleep and Weight-Related Hormones

1. Leptin and Ghrelin Regulation

Leptin Production: Adequate sleep supports the production of leptin, signaling satiety and reducing the desire to eat.

Ghrelin Levels: Sleep deprivation increases ghrelin levels, leading to increased hunger and a preference for high-calorie foods.

2. Cortisol and Stress-Related Weight Changes

Cortisol Regulation: Lack of sleep may elevate cortisol levels, promoting fat storage and contributing to stress-related weight changes.

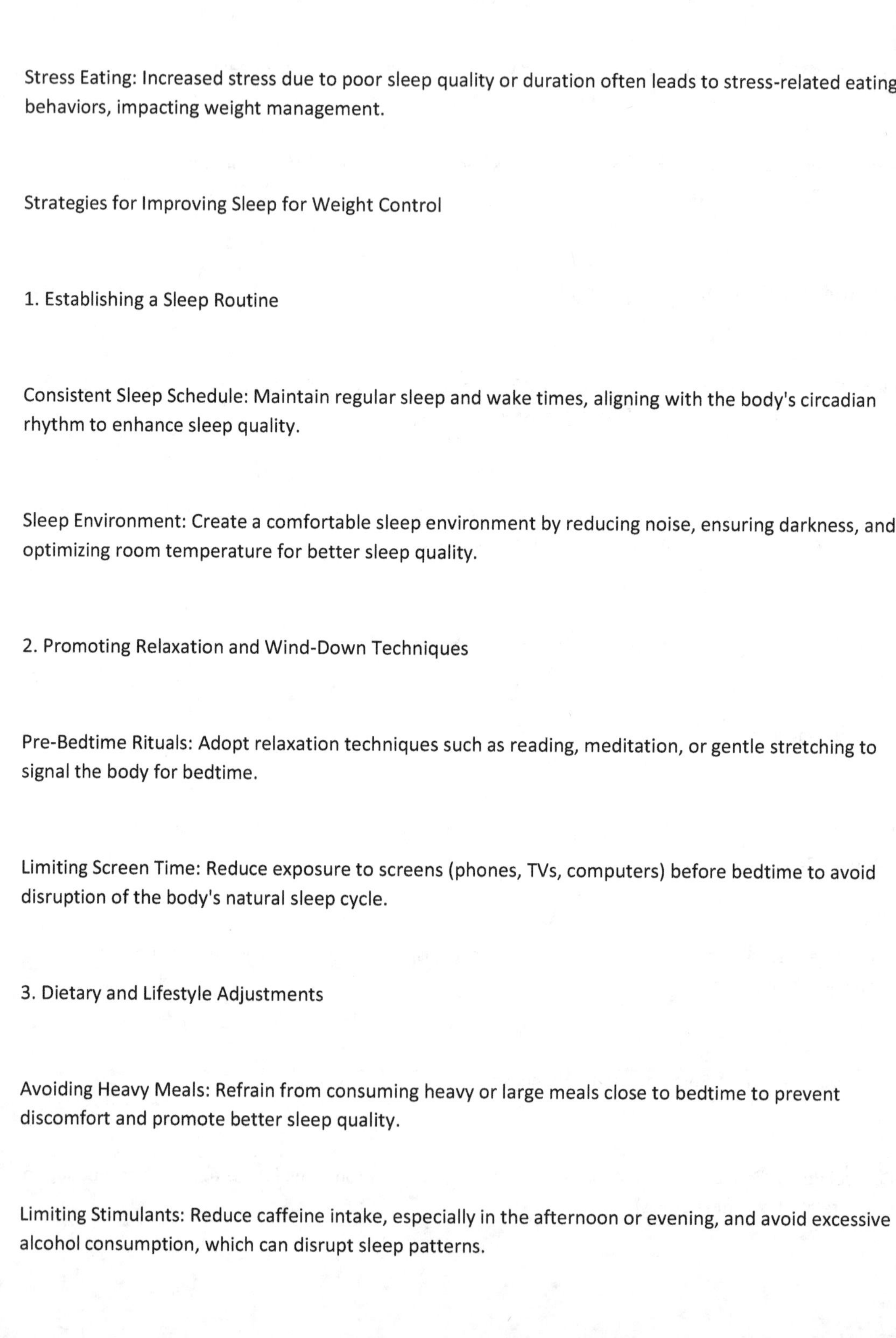

Stress Eating: Increased stress due to poor sleep quality or duration often leads to stress-related eating behaviors, impacting weight management.

Strategies for Improving Sleep for Weight Control

1. Establishing a Sleep Routine

Consistent Sleep Schedule: Maintain regular sleep and wake times, aligning with the body's circadian rhythm to enhance sleep quality.

Sleep Environment: Create a comfortable sleep environment by reducing noise, ensuring darkness, and optimizing room temperature for better sleep quality.

2. Promoting Relaxation and Wind-Down Techniques

Pre-Bedtime Rituals: Adopt relaxation techniques such as reading, meditation, or gentle stretching to signal the body for bedtime.

Limiting Screen Time: Reduce exposure to screens (phones, TVs, computers) before bedtime to avoid disruption of the body's natural sleep cycle.

3. Dietary and Lifestyle Adjustments

Avoiding Heavy Meals: Refrain from consuming heavy or large meals close to bedtime to prevent discomfort and promote better sleep quality.

Limiting Stimulants: Reduce caffeine intake, especially in the afternoon or evening, and avoid excessive alcohol consumption, which can disrupt sleep patterns.

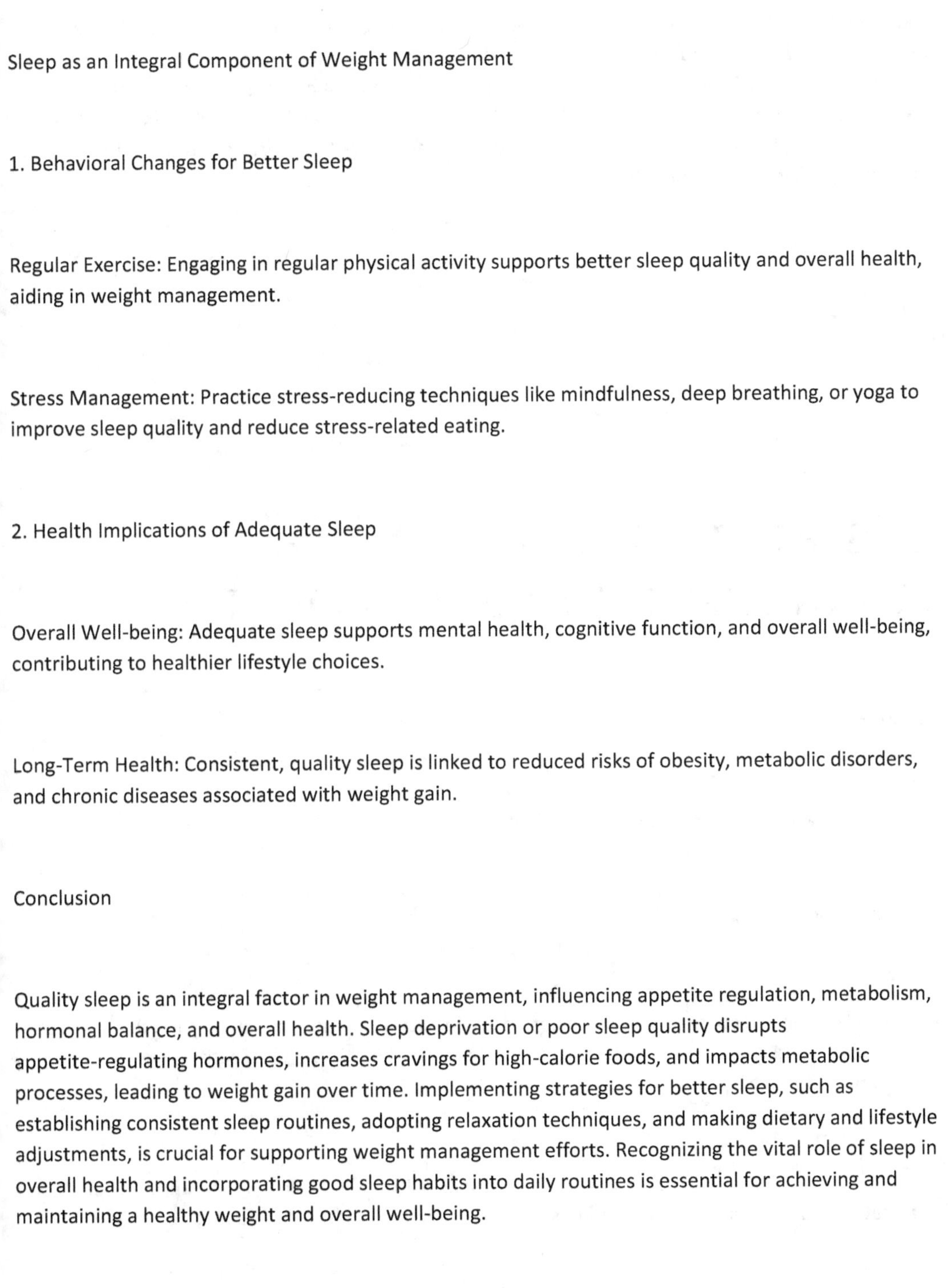

Sleep as an Integral Component of Weight Management

1. Behavioral Changes for Better Sleep

Regular Exercise: Engaging in regular physical activity supports better sleep quality and overall health, aiding in weight management.

Stress Management: Practice stress-reducing techniques like mindfulness, deep breathing, or yoga to improve sleep quality and reduce stress-related eating.

2. Health Implications of Adequate Sleep

Overall Well-being: Adequate sleep supports mental health, cognitive function, and overall well-being, contributing to healthier lifestyle choices.

Long-Term Health: Consistent, quality sleep is linked to reduced risks of obesity, metabolic disorders, and chronic diseases associated with weight gain.

Conclusion

Quality sleep is an integral factor in weight management, influencing appetite regulation, metabolism, hormonal balance, and overall health. Sleep deprivation or poor sleep quality disrupts appetite-regulating hormones, increases cravings for high-calorie foods, and impacts metabolic processes, leading to weight gain over time. Implementing strategies for better sleep, such as establishing consistent sleep routines, adopting relaxation techniques, and making dietary and lifestyle adjustments, is crucial for supporting weight management efforts. Recognizing the vital role of sleep in overall health and incorporating good sleep habits into daily routines is essential for achieving and maintaining a healthy weight and overall well-being.

Understanding the intricate connection between sleep and weight management underscores the importance of prioritizing quality sleep for overall health. Implementing strategies to improve sleep quality, establish consistent sleep routines, and adopt relaxation techniques supports weight management efforts by influencing appetite regulation, metabolism, and hormonal balance. Embracing healthy sleep habits as an integral part of a holistic approach to wellness fosters better health outcomes and aids in sustainable weight management.

UNDERSTANDING WEIGHT MANAGEMENT: 2024 EDITION

CHAPTER 5

Understanding the Connection Between Sleep and Weight

1. Hormonal Regulation and Appetite

Leptin and Ghrelin: Sleep influences these hormones, impacting hunger and satiety cues. Inadequate sleep disrupts leptin (suppresses appetite) and increases ghrelin (stimulates appetite), leading to overeating and weight gain.

Insulin Sensitivity: Poor sleep patterns affect insulin sensitivity, contributing to imbalances in blood sugar levels and potential weight-related issues like insulin resistance and metabolic disruptions.

2. Metabolic Rate and Energy Balance

Metabolism and Sleep: Inadequate sleep affects metabolic rate and energy expenditure, potentially leading to weight gain by disrupting the body's ability to process and utilize energy efficiently.

Physical Activity Levels: Fatigue from lack of sleep may reduce motivation for physical activity, impacting overall energy expenditure and hindering weight management efforts.

Strategies for Improving Sleep Quality for Weight Control

1. Creating an Optimal Sleep Environment

Comfortable Sleep Setup: Ensure a conducive sleep environment, including a comfortable mattress, appropriate room temperature, and minimal disruptions for better sleep quality.

Light and Noise Control: Minimize exposure to light and noise during bedtime by using blackout curtains and white noise machines to promote deeper and uninterrupted sleep.

2. Establishing Consistent Sleep Habits

Sleep Schedule: Maintain a regular sleep-wake cycle, aiming for the recommended 7-9 hours of sleep per night, aligning with the body's circadian rhythm for better sleep quality.

Bedtime Rituals: Adopt relaxing bedtime routines, such as reading, taking a warm bath, or practicing relaxation techniques to signal the body for sleep.

3. Diet and Lifestyle Adjustments for Better Sleep

Mindful Eating: Avoid heavy or large meals close to bedtime, opting for lighter, easily digestible snacks if necessary to prevent discomfort and promote better sleep quality.

Limiting Stimulants: Reduce caffeine intake, especially in the afternoon or evening, and minimize alcohol consumption, both of which can disrupt sleep patterns and affect sleep quality.

Importance of Consistent Sleep Patterns for Weight Management

1. Impact on Appetite Regulation

Hormonal Balance: Consistent sleep patterns support hormonal balance, aiding in the regulation of leptin and ghrelin, thereby controlling appetite and reducing cravings.

Stress and Emotional Eating: Better sleep quality reduces stress levels, minimizing stress-related eating behaviors and promoting healthier dietary choices conducive to weight control.

2. Metabolic Health and Weight Control

Enhanced Metabolism: Consistent sleep supports metabolic health, optimizing the body's ability to process energy efficiently and promoting weight management.

Improved Physical Performance: Quality sleep enhances physical performance, motivation for exercise, and overall energy levels, supporting consistent physical activity for weight control.

Holistic Approach to Sleep for Effective Weight Management

1. Behavioral Changes for Better Sleep

Regular Exercise: Engaging in regular physical activity promotes better sleep quality and contributes to overall health and weight management efforts.

Stress Management: Stress-reducing practices like meditation, deep breathing, or yoga support better sleep patterns, reducing stress-related eating and aiding weight control.

2. Health Implications of Consistent Sleep

Cognitive Function: Adequate sleep improves cognitive function, concentration, and decision-making abilities, aiding in making healthier lifestyle choices, including dietary habits.

Long-Term Health: Consistent, quality sleep is associated with reduced risks of obesity, chronic diseases, and improved overall health, highlighting its importance in weight management and well-being.

Conclusion

The relationship between sleep and weight is intricate, impacting hormonal regulation, appetite control, metabolism, and overall health. Implementing strategies to improve sleep quality, establishing consistent sleep patterns, and adopting healthier lifestyle habits play pivotal roles in weight management efforts. Recognizing the significance of consistent sleep for hormonal balance, metabolic health, and improved cognitive function underscores the importance of prioritizing quality sleep as a fundamental pillar of effective weight control. Embracing holistic approaches to enhance sleep quality promotes better health outcomes, aiding in sustainable weight management and overall well-being.

Understanding the critical link between sleep and weight management highlights the importance of adopting strategies to improve sleep quality and establish consistent sleep patterns. Prioritizing quality sleep aids in hormonal regulation, appetite control, metabolic balance, and overall health, supporting effective weight management efforts. By incorporating healthy sleep habits into daily routines, individuals can enhance their overall well-being and achieve sustainable weight control, emphasizing the pivotal role of consistent, quality sleep in maintaining a healthy lifestyle.

Stress and Its Influence on Weight

1. Hormonal Response to Stress

Cortisol Release: Stress triggers the release of cortisol, the primary stress hormone, impacting appetite regulation, metabolism, and fat storage.

Increased Cravings: Elevated cortisol levels often lead to increased cravings for high-calorie, high-sugar foods, contributing to weight gain.

2. Emotional Eating and Stress

Comfort Eating: Stress often triggers emotional eating behaviors, leading individuals to seek comfort in food as a coping mechanism, which may result in overeating and weight gain.

Mindless Eating: Stress may cause individuals to engage in mindless eating, leading to poor food choices and an increased intake of unhealthy, calorie-dense foods.

Impact of Stress on Metabolism and Weight Control

1. Metabolic Changes Due to Stress

Metabolism Disruption: Chronic stress may disrupt metabolic processes, leading to an increase in fat accumulation, particularly around the abdominal area.

Slowed Digestion: Stress can impact digestive processes, leading to slowed digestion and potential weight-related issues.

2. Sleep Disturbances and Weight Management

Stress and Sleep Quality: Chronic stress often leads to sleep disturbances, affecting sleep quality and duration, which can contribute to weight gain over time.

Impact on Hormones: Poor sleep patterns due to stress may disrupt hormonal balance, affecting appetite-regulating hormones and metabolism.

Strategies for Managing Stress for Weight Control

1. Stress-Reducing Techniques

Mindfulness Practices: Incorporate mindfulness, meditation, deep breathing exercises, or yoga to reduce stress levels and promote relaxation.

Physical Activity: Engage in regular exercise, which acts as a stress-reliever, aiding in reducing cortisol levels and supporting overall well-being.

2. Healthy Coping Mechanisms

Stress Management Skills: Develop effective stress management skills such as time management, setting boundaries, and seeking social support to mitigate stressors.

Positive Outlets: Engage in hobbies, activities, or creative outlets that provide stress relief and serve as healthy distractions from stress-induced eating.

Behavioral Changes for Stress Reduction and Weight Management

1. Mindful Eating Practices

Awareness of Triggers: Recognize stress-related triggers for emotional eating and practice mindfulness to address and cope with these triggers without resorting to food.

Healthy Food Choices: Opt for nutrient-dense, whole foods when stressed instead of high-calorie, processed foods to manage stress-induced cravings.

2. Promoting Emotional Well-being

Self-Care Practices: Prioritize self-care, adequate rest, and relaxation techniques to reduce stress levels and promote emotional well-being.

Seeking Support: Seek professional help or counseling to manage stress effectively and develop coping strategies that do not involve overeating.

Importance of Stress Management for Weight Control

1. Long-Term Health Implications

Stress Reduction and Health: Managing stress effectively supports long-term health by reducing the risk of obesity, metabolic disorders, and chronic diseases associated with weight gain.

Holistic Approach to Weight Management: Stress management is a crucial aspect of a holistic approach to weight control, supporting behavioral changes and healthy lifestyle habits.

2. Behavioral Modifications for Sustainable Weight Management

Consistency in Stress Management: Consistent stress management practices aid in sustaining healthy eating behaviors and overall weight control efforts.

Mind-Body Connection: Understanding the connection between stress and weight helps in adopting holistic approaches that prioritize emotional well-being alongside physical health.

Conclusion

The impact of stress on weight is significant, influencing eating behaviors, metabolism, and overall health. Stress triggers hormonal responses that impact appetite, increase cravings, and disrupt metabolism, contributing to weight gain. Implementing stress management strategies, such as mindfulness practices, healthy coping mechanisms, and engaging in physical activity, plays a pivotal role in weight control efforts. Recognizing the importance of stress management as an integral part of a holistic approach to weight management underscores the need for adopting healthy stress-reducing behaviors and fostering emotional well-being. By prioritizing stress management, individuals can support healthy eating habits, promote weight control, and enhance overall health and well-being.

Understanding the impact of stress on weight highlights the significance of stress management in effective weight control. Implementing stress-reducing strategies and healthy coping mechanisms aids in mitigating stress-induced eating behaviors, supporting better dietary choices, and promoting overall well-being. By prioritizing stress management as part of a holistic approach to health, individuals can foster healthier lifestyle habits, leading to sustainable weight management and improved quality of life.

Impact of Stress on Weight Gain

1. Hormonal Changes and Appetite Regulation

Cortisol and Appetite: Elevated cortisol levels from chronic stress can disrupt appetite regulation, leading to increased cravings for high-calorie foods.

Emotional Eating: Stress often triggers emotional eating behaviors, encouraging individuals to seek comfort in food, potentially resulting in overeating and weight gain.

2. Metabolic Alterations Due to Stress

Metabolism Disruption: Prolonged stress may disrupt metabolic processes, leading to increased fat accumulation and potential weight-related issues.

Sleep Disturbances: Stress-induced sleep disturbances can impact hormonal balance and appetite-regulating hormones, affecting weight management.

Techniques for Stress Reduction and Weight Maintenance

1. Stress-Relieving Activities

Physical Exercise: Engage in regular physical activity, which acts as a stress-reliever, reducing cortisol levels and aiding in weight maintenance.

Mindfulness Practices: Incorporate mindfulness, meditation, or yoga to reduce stress levels, promoting relaxation and aiding weight management efforts.

2. Healthy Coping Mechanisms

Stress Management Skills: Develop effective stress management skills such as time management, setting boundaries, and seeking social support to mitigate stressors.

Positive Outlets: Cultivate hobbies, activities, or creative outlets as healthy distractions from stress-induced eating, fostering emotional well-being.

Mindfulness and Its Role in Managing Weight-Related Stress

1. Mindful Eating Practices

Stress Awareness: Practice mindfulness to recognize stress-induced eating triggers and adopt healthier coping mechanisms instead of turning to food.

Conscious Food Choices: Opt for nutrient-dense, whole foods over high-calorie, processed options when experiencing stress to manage cravings.

2. Promoting Emotional Well-being

Self-Care and Rest: Prioritize self-care, adequate rest, and relaxation techniques to reduce stress levels, promoting emotional well-being and weight control.

Professional Support: Seek professional help or counseling to manage stress effectively and develop coping strategies for stress-related weight gain.

Understanding the Mind-Body Connection in Stress Management

1. Stress-Weight Relationship

Holistic Approach: Understanding the mind-body connection aids in adopting a holistic approach to stress management and weight control.

Consistent Stress Management: Consistency in stress management practices supports healthier eating habits and sustainable weight management efforts.

2. Mindfulness and Stress Reduction

Mindfulness Techniques: Practicing mindfulness helps in stress reduction, promoting healthier responses to stressors, and aiding in weight maintenance.

Emotional Regulation: Mindfulness techniques enable better emotional regulation, reducing the likelihood of stress-induced eating behaviors.

Conclusion

The impact of stress on weight gain is multifaceted, influencing hormonal responses, appetite regulation, and metabolic processes. Chronic stress often leads to emotional eating behaviors, disruptions in metabolism, and sleep disturbances, contributing to weight gain over time. Adopting stress reduction techniques, practicing mindfulness, and cultivating healthy coping mechanisms play crucial roles in mitigating stress-induced weight gain. Recognizing the mind-body connection and employing mindfulness practices aids in managing stress-related eating behaviors, promoting emotional well-being, and supporting weight maintenance efforts. By prioritizing stress reduction as part of a holistic approach to health, individuals can foster healthier lifestyles, enhance weight control, and improve overall well-being.

Understanding the complex interplay between stress and weight gain underscores the importance of stress management techniques in maintaining a healthy weight. Incorporating stress reduction strategies, practicing mindfulness, and nurturing healthy coping mechanisms help mitigate stress-induced eating behaviors, contributing to improved weight management and emotional well-being. Embracing mindfulness practices and recognizing the mind-body connection supports healthier responses to stress, aiding in weight maintenance and fostering overall health and wellness.

Importance of Long-Term Strategies in Weight Maintenance

1. Mindset Shift for Sustainable Changes

Lifestyle Transformation: Transitioning from short-term diets to long-term lifestyle changes fosters a sustainable approach to weight management.

Behavioral Adaptations: Embrace a mindset centered on gradual, consistent changes rather than quick fixes for long-term success.

2. Habits and Behavioral Adjustments

Building Healthy Habits: Establishing sustainable habits around nutrition, exercise, stress management, and sleep promotes lasting weight control.

Behavioral Modification: Implementing behavior-focused strategies aids in maintaining weight loss, emphasizing consistency and self-awareness.

Nutritional Strategies for Long-Term Weight Management

1. Balanced and Sustainable Diet

Whole Foods Emphasis: Prioritize nutrient-dense whole foods while allowing occasional indulgences to sustain healthy eating habits.

Portion Control: Practice mindful eating and portion control, focusing on quality and quantity to maintain a balanced diet.

2. Regular Monitoring and Adaptation

Periodic Assessments: Regularly monitor dietary intake, reassess goals, and make necessary adjustments to accommodate lifestyle changes and prevent stagnation.

Flexibility and Adaptability: Embrace flexibility in diet plans, incorporating diverse foods and making adjustments without compromising health.

Exercise and Physical Activity for Long-Term Health

1. Sustainable Exercise Routines

Diverse Workouts: Engage in a variety of physical activities to prevent boredom, promote adherence, and continually challenge the body.

Consistency over Intensity: Prioritize consistency in exercise routines rather than extreme intensity, focusing on regular movement for sustainable results.

2. Integration of Daily Movement

Active Lifestyle: Incorporate daily movement, such as walking, taking the stairs, or stretching, to complement structured workouts and promote an active lifestyle.

Incorporating Strength Training: Integrate resistance training to maintain muscle mass, support metabolism, and enhance overall physical strength.

Behavioral and Lifestyle Adjustments for Maintenance

1. Stress Reduction and Emotional Well-being

Stress Management: Prioritize stress reduction through mindfulness, relaxation techniques, and healthy coping mechanisms to mitigate stress-related weight gain.

Emotional Regulation: Practice emotional resilience, learning to manage emotions without resorting to emotional eating, fostering better control over eating habits.

2. Consistent Sleep Patterns

Prioritizing Quality Sleep: Maintain consistent sleep schedules, ensuring adequate sleep duration and quality, which aids in hormonal balance and weight management.

Sleep Hygiene Practices: Implement sleep hygiene routines, creating optimal sleep environments conducive to restorative sleep for overall health.

Strategies for Behavioral Adherence and Long-Term Success

1. Accountability and Support Systems

Accountability Partners: Seek support from friends, family, or support groups to stay accountable and motivated on the weight management journey.

Professional Guidance: Work with health professionals, nutritionists, or trainers for guidance, motivation, and strategies tailored to individual needs.

2. Mindfulness and Holistic Wellness

Mindful Practices: Embrace mindfulness in daily life, practicing mindful eating, stress reduction, and self-awareness to maintain a balanced approach to health.

Holistic Wellness Approach: Focus on overall wellness, emphasizing mental, emotional, and physical health for sustained weight management and well-being.

Conclusion

Long-term weight management involves embracing sustainable strategies that encompass dietary changes, regular physical activity, stress reduction, and holistic well-being. Shifting from short-term solutions to lifestyle modifications facilitates lasting weight control. Establishing healthy habits, monitoring progress, and making adaptive changes over time form the foundation for sustained success. Incorporating balanced nutrition, regular exercise, stress management, consistent sleep patterns, and mindful practices fosters a holistic approach to maintaining weight loss and overall wellness. Long-term success in weight maintenance necessitates a commitment to lifelong behavioral changes, creating a sustainable, healthy lifestyle.

Long-term weight management necessitates a commitment to sustainable habits, behavioral adjustments, and a balanced approach to nutrition, exercise, stress management, and overall well-being. By embracing lasting strategies and making gradual, consistent changes, individuals can maintain weight loss, promote overall health, and sustain a healthier lifestyle for the long term. Implementing these strategies forms the cornerstone of a successful and fulfilling journey towards sustained weight management and improved well-being.

Understanding Sustainable Weight Loss

1. Lifestyle Modification over Short-Term Fixes

Behavioral Changes: Embrace lifestyle modifications focusing on dietary changes, increased physical activity, and stress reduction for sustainable weight loss.

Mindset Shift: Adopt a long-term mindset, prioritizing health and well-being over rapid weight loss, to ensure lasting results.

Nutritional Strategies for Sustainable Weight Loss

1. Balanced and Nutrient-Dense Diet

Whole Foods Emphasis: Prioritize whole, unprocessed foods rich in nutrients, fibers, and healthy fats, while minimizing processed and high-sugar foods.

Portion Control: Practice mindful eating, paying attention to portion sizes, and savoring meals to prevent overeating and foster better digestion.

2. Meal Planning and Consistency

Regular Meal Patterns: Establish consistent eating patterns, including regular meals and snacks, to maintain energy levels and prevent excessive hunger.

Meal Prepping: Plan and prepare meals in advance to ensure healthier food choices and avoid impulsive, unhealthy eating decisions.

Exercise and Physical Activity for Sustainable Weight Loss

1. Regular Physical Activity

Variety in Workouts: Engage in diverse exercises that suit personal preferences, promoting enjoyment and sustainability in fitness routines.

Incremental Progress: Gradually increase exercise intensity or duration over time, focusing on consistency rather than extreme workouts.

2. Incorporating Daily Movement

Active Lifestyle: Embrace daily movement, such as walking, cycling, or taking the stairs, to complement structured workouts and increase overall activity levels.

Strength Training: Include resistance or strength training to build muscle, support metabolism, and enhance overall physical fitness.

Behavioral Changes and Mindfulness

1. Stress Management for Weight Loss

Stress Reduction Techniques: Incorporate stress-relieving activities like meditation, yoga, or deep breathing to minimize stress-induced eating.

Coping Strategies: Develop healthy coping mechanisms to address stress without resorting to emotional eating, ensuring better control over food choices.

2. Quality Sleep and Emotional Well-being

Sleep Hygiene: Prioritize adequate sleep and establish good sleep hygiene practices, as sleep influences hormones regulating appetite and metabolism.

Emotional Regulation: Enhance emotional resilience and mindfulness, fostering a healthier relationship with food and improving overall well-being.

Support Systems and Accountability

1. Seeking Support and Guidance

Professional Assistance: Consult with healthcare professionals, dietitians, or fitness trainers for personalized guidance and support tailored to individual needs.

Community Engagement: Join support groups or online communities to share experiences, seek motivation, and stay accountable on the weight loss journey.

2. Tracking and Monitoring Progress

Recording Progress: Keep track of food intake, exercise routines, and emotional well-being to monitor progress and make necessary adjustments.

Celebrating Milestones: Celebrate achievements and milestones, no matter how small, to stay motivated and reinforce positive behavioral changes.

Conclusion

Sustainable weight loss entails adopting a holistic approach that emphasizes balanced nutrition, regular exercise, stress reduction, and behavioral modifications. It involves making gradual, consistent changes in lifestyle rather than resorting to quick-fix solutions. By prioritizing whole foods, portion control, regular physical activity, stress management, and support systems, individuals can achieve sustainable weight loss and maintain a healthier lifestyle. Incorporating these sustainable strategies fosters not only weight loss but also overall well-being and long-term health.

Sustainable weight loss strategies encompass a balanced approach involving dietary changes, regular physical activity, stress management, and behavioral adjustments. By embracing these sustainable practices and making gradual lifestyle modifications, individuals can achieve lasting weight loss and improved overall health. The focus on balanced nutrition, consistent exercise, stress reduction, and seeking support systems ensures not just weight loss but the maintenance of a healthier and more fulfilling lifestyle in the long term.

UNDERSTANDING WEIGHT MANAGEMENT: 2024 EDITION

CHAPTER 6

Building Healthy Habits for Long-Term Weight Management

1. Consistent and Balanced Nutrition

Whole Foods Emphasis: Prioritize nutrient-dense whole foods, fruits, vegetables, lean proteins, and healthy fats in daily meals for sustained energy and satiety.

Mindful Eating: Cultivate mindful eating habits by paying attention to hunger cues, practicing portion control, and savoring meals to prevent overeating.

2. Regular Physical Activity and Exercise

Variety in Workouts: Engage in diverse exercises or activities that you enjoy, ensuring consistency and preventing boredom, promoting adherence to a regular routine.

Incorporating Daily Movement: Embrace an active lifestyle by integrating small bursts of movement throughout the day, like walking, stretching breaks, or taking stairs.

Strategies to Prevent Weight Regain

1. Continuous Behavior Monitoring

Regular Self-Assessment: Continuously monitor eating behaviors, physical activity levels, and emotional well-being to identify triggers for weight regain.

Adjusting Habits: Make necessary adjustments in diet or exercise routines to counteract any weight fluctuations and prevent regression into unhealthy patterns.

2. Sustaining Lifestyle Changes

Long-Term Mindset: Adopt a permanent lifestyle change mentality, viewing weight management as an ongoing journey rather than a short-term goal.

Consistency in Habits: Maintain consistency in healthy eating, regular exercise, and stress management to prevent relapse into previous behaviors.

Balancing Lifestyle Changes with Social Life and Celebrations

1. Mindful Decision-Making in Social Settings

Prioritizing Healthy Choices: Opt for healthier options when dining out or attending social gatherings, focusing on portion control and nutrient-rich foods.

Navigating Temptations: Develop strategies to manage temptations and peer influence without compromising healthy habits, such as planning ahead or setting limits.

2. Celebrating Without Compromise

Flexible Approaches: Embrace flexible eating habits during celebrations, allowing indulgence in moderation without guilt while compensating with healthier choices later.

Active Celebrations: Incorporate physical activities or fun outings into celebratory events, promoting movement and making them more than just food-centric occasions.

Integrating Lifestyle Changes into Social Interactions

1. Communicating Healthy Choices

Open Communication: Communicate personal health goals with friends and family to garner support and encourage healthier options in social settings.

Setting Boundaries: Establish boundaries regarding food choices and portions, ensuring adherence to healthy habits without feeling pressured to overindulge.

2. Creating Healthy Social Activities

Active Outings: Organize activities centered around physical movement, like group hikes, dance classes, or sports, fostering a healthier social environment.

Health-Focused Gatherings: Host gatherings emphasizing healthier food choices or cooking sessions, encouraging friends and family to engage in nutritious eating.

Conclusion

Building healthy habits for long-term weight management involves consistent efforts in nutrition, physical activity, and lifestyle adjustments. Strategies to prevent weight regain revolve around continuous monitoring, sustaining healthy habits, and adapting to changes over time. Balancing lifestyle changes with social life and celebrations requires mindfulness, communication, and the incorporation of healthy choices into social interactions without compromising enjoyment. By integrating these strategies, individuals can maintain a healthy weight while enjoying social occasions, ensuring sustainable habits for long-term weight management.

Building healthy habits for long-term weight management requires consistency, mindfulness, and flexibility in incorporating lifestyle changes. Strategies to prevent weight regain involve continuous monitoring, lifestyle adjustments, and maintaining a long-term mindset. Balancing lifestyle changes with social interactions and celebrations necessitates mindful decision-making, open communication, and the incorporation of healthy choices without compromising enjoyment. By integrating these strategies, individuals can maintain a healthy weight while enjoying social occasions, ensuring sustained habits for long-term weight management and overall well-being.

Importance of Tracking Progress in Weight Management

1. Monitoring Physical Changes

Regular Measurements: Tracking body weight, measurements, or body composition changes helps monitor progress accurately over time.

Visual Records: Taking progress photos provides visual cues of changes in physique, offering motivation and insight into the transformation.

2. Behavioral Monitoring

Food Diary: Keeping a food journal aids in understanding eating patterns, identifying triggers, and making informed dietary adjustments.

Activity Logs: Recording exercise routines or daily activities helps evaluate consistency and make necessary modifications.

Setting Realistic and Achievable Goals

1. SMART Goal Setting

Specific: Define clear, precise objectives, such as losing a specific amount of weight or improving fitness levels.

Measurable: Set quantifiable parameters to track progress effectively, enabling measurement and adjustment.

2. Adaptable and Realistic Goals

Achievability: Ensure goals are attainable within a reasonable time frame, considering lifestyle, resources, and individual capabilities.

Flexibility: Remain open to adjusting goals as circumstances change, allowing for realistic expectations and preventing discouragement.

Strategies for Adjusting Goals

1. Evaluating Progress and Assessing Results

Regular Assessments: Reassess goals periodically, analyzing progress against set benchmarks to determine if adjustments are needed.

Reviewing Successes and Challenges: Identify what has worked and what needs improvement, learning from successes and setbacks.

2. Modifying Approaches and Strategies

Changing Methods: Adapt dietary plans or workout routines if progress stalls, incorporating new techniques or intensifying workouts.

Gradual Adjustments: Make gradual changes to goals, considering small tweaks to enhance progress without overwhelming changes.

Adapting Strategies for Long-Term Success

1. Behavioral Modifications

Lifestyle Adjustments: Focus on sustainable changes, altering habits slowly for long-term adherence rather than drastic, short-lived transformations.

Mindful Eating Practices: Practice mindful eating, incorporating healthier food choices into daily routines for lasting dietary changes.

2. Continuous Learning and Improvement

Education and Awareness: Stay informed about nutrition, exercise, and wellness trends, implementing new knowledge for continual improvement.

Seeking Support: Consult with professionals or join support groups for guidance, motivation, and accountability in achieving goals.

Balancing Persistence and Adaptability

1. Maintaining Motivation

Celebrating Milestones: Acknowledge and celebrate achievements along the journey, reinforcing positive behaviors and sustaining motivation.

Mindset Maintenance: Cultivate a positive mindset, understanding that setbacks are part of the process, and perseverance is key to long-term success.

2. Staying Consistent with Adjustments

Consistent Efforts: Continue efforts even during plateaus, knowing that adjustments take time to yield results and persistence is fundamental.

Tracking Adaptations: Monitor the effects of goal adjustments and strategies, ensuring they align with desired outcomes.

Conclusion

Tracking progress and adjusting goals are essential components of successful weight management. By regularly monitoring physical changes, setting realistic goals, and adapting strategies, individuals can achieve sustainable progress. It's crucial to set achievable goals, regularly assess progress, and modify approaches as needed. Balancing persistence with adaptability ensures long-term success in weight management. Consistent efforts, gradual modifications, and maintaining a positive mindset are fundamental to achieving and maintaining health and wellness goals.

Tracking progress and adjusting goals are fundamental to successful weight management. Consistent monitoring, realistic goal setting, and adapting strategies are key for sustainable progress. Balancing persistence with adaptability ensures long-term success in weight management, fostering a healthier lifestyle and improved overall well-being. These practices allow individuals to navigate their weight management journey effectively, making necessary adjustments while staying committed to achieving and maintaining their health goals.

Importance of Monitoring Progress in Weight Management

1. Tracking Physical Changes

Measurement of Body Metrics: Regularly monitoring weight, body measurements, and body fat percentage helps gauge progress accurately.

Observing Changes: Tracking changes in appearance, clothing fit, and muscle tone provides tangible indicators of progress.

2. Behavioral Observations

Dietary Tracking: Keeping a food diary aids in understanding eating habits, identifying patterns, and making necessary dietary adjustments.

Exercise Monitoring: Recording exercise routines, duration, and intensity helps ensure consistency and adherence to fitness goals.

Using Technology for Tracking and Analyzing Data

1. Utilizing Fitness Apps and Devices

Activity Trackers: Wearable devices or smartphone apps monitor steps, heart rate, and calories burned, providing real-time data on physical activity.

Nutrition Apps: Food tracking apps help log meals, count calories, and analyze macronutrient intake for better dietary management.

2. Data Analysis and Insights

Data Visualization: Tools that visualize progress through graphs or charts offer a clear representation of trends, aiding in goal assessment.

Analyzing Trends: Technology allows for analyzing trends in eating, exercise, and weight changes, providing insights for adjustments.

Strategies for Adjusting Goals and Staying Motivated

1. Goal Adjustment Techniques

Regular Evaluations: Periodically review progress against set goals, making adjustments based on current achievements and challenges.

Realistic Modifications: Modify goals to align with evolving circumstances, ensuring they remain achievable and motivating.

2. Maintaining Motivation

Positive Reinforcement: Celebrate milestones, whether big or small, to boost motivation and reinforce positive behaviors.

Visual Progress Tracking: Utilize progress photos or visual representations to see tangible improvements, fostering continued dedication.

Staying Motivated and Goal-Oriented

1. Creating Accountability

Accountability Partnerships: Partner with friends or join support groups for mutual motivation, encouragement, and accountability.

Professional Support: Seek guidance from health professionals or fitness coaches for expert advice and encouragement.

2. Mindset and Behavioral Modifications

Mindfulness Practices: Practice mindfulness techniques to stay focused on present goals, reducing stress, and aiding in decision-making.

Habit Formation: Cultivate healthier habits gradually, reinforcing positive behaviors to ensure sustained progress.

Balancing Technology and Personal Motivation

1. Technology as a Motivational Tool

Visualizing Progress: Technology offers visual representations of progress, motivating individuals to continue their efforts.

Enhanced Monitoring: Detailed data tracking through technology provides a clearer understanding of trends, fostering motivation to improve.

2. Maintaining Intrinsic Motivation

Internal Rewards: Cultivate internal motivation by focusing on the intrinsic benefits of improved health and well-being.

Consistency in Habits: Establishing consistent healthy habits independent of technology ensures lasting behavioral changes.

Conclusion

Monitoring progress in weight management is integral to achieving and sustaining success. Leveraging technology for data tracking and analysis provides valuable insights and motivation. Adjusting goals based on monitored progress ensures they remain realistic and achievable. Staying motivated involves a combination of positive reinforcement, mindfulness, accountability, and a focus on intrinsic rewards. Balancing the benefits of technology with personal motivation is key to maintaining consistency in healthy habits and achieving long-term success in weight management.

Monitoring progress in weight management is a crucial component of achieving and maintaining success. Technology plays a vital role in tracking data, providing insights, and motivating individuals throughout their journey. Adjusting goals based on progress ensures they remain realistic and achievable. Staying motivated involves a combination of positive reinforcement, mindfulness, and accountability. Balancing the benefits of technology with personal motivation is essential for consistency in healthy habits and sustained success in weight management.

Special Considerations in Weight Management

1. Age-related Considerations

Metabolism Changes: Metabolic rate tends to decrease with age, requiring adjustments in dietary intake and exercise to maintain weight.

Bone Health: Older adults should focus on adequate nutrition and weight-bearing exercises to support bone health and prevent osteoporosis.

2. Gender-specific Challenges

Hormonal Influence: Hormonal differences may impact weight loss and gain differently among genders, requiring personalized approaches.

Pregnancy and Postpartum: Addressing weight concerns during and after pregnancy involves specialized considerations for healthy weight management.

Health Conditions and Weight Management

1. Medical Considerations

Chronic Conditions: Managing weight alongside conditions like diabetes or heart disease requires tailored dietary and exercise plans under medical supervision.

Medications and Weight: Some medications may impact weight, requiring adjustments in diet or exercise routines.

2. Mental Health and Weight

Emotional Eating: Addressing mental health concerns like anxiety or depression is crucial to avoid emotional eating patterns.

Stress Management: Developing coping mechanisms to manage stress effectively aids in preventing stress-induced weight fluctuations.

Socio-cultural Factors and Challenges

1. Cultural Influences

Dietary Preferences: Adapting dietary changes considering cultural food preferences or restrictions is essential for adherence.

Social Norms: Navigating social gatherings or events where food plays a significant role can pose challenges in maintaining healthy eating habits.

2. Economic Considerations

Food Accessibility: Access to healthy and affordable food options may be limited, requiring creative strategies to maintain a nutritious diet.

Resource Constraints: Financial limitations might affect access to fitness facilities or resources, demanding alternative affordable exercise options.

Challenges Faced in Weight Management

1. Plateaus and Setbacks

Weight Plateaus: Stagnation in weight loss progress might occur, necessitating adjustments in diet or exercise routines.

Dealing with Setbacks: Addressing setbacks or relapses in habits requires resilience and strategies to regain momentum.

2. Motivation and Adherence

Lack of Motivation: Maintaining long-term motivation requires consistent reinforcement and adaptability in goals.

Adherence to Changes: Sustaining lifestyle modifications demands commitment, often facing challenges due to routine disruptions or lack of consistency.

Strategies to Address Special Considerations and Challenges

1. Personalized Approaches

Consulting Professionals: Seeking guidance from healthcare providers or nutritionists aids in creating personalized plans considering individual needs.

Adaptable Strategies: Flexibility in adjusting plans based on special considerations or challenges ensures ongoing progress.

2. Mindfulness and Resilience Building

Mindful Practices: Incorporating mindfulness techniques aids in managing stress, emotions, and making mindful food choices.

Building Resilience: Cultivating resilience helps individuals bounce back from setbacks, fostering a positive mindset towards long-term goals.

Conclusion

Navigating the complexities and challenges in weight management involves addressing special considerations such as age-related changes, health conditions, socio-cultural influences, and various hurdles encountered during the journey. Strategies tailored to individual needs, considering medical conditions, cultural influences, and economic constraints, are crucial for successful weight management. Moreover, fostering resilience, adapting personalized approaches, and maintaining mindfulness play pivotal roles in overcoming challenges and achieving sustainable weight management.

Special considerations and challenges in weight management encompass various factors like age, health conditions, socio-cultural influences, and personal hurdles. Addressing these factors through personalized approaches, resilience-building strategies, and mindfulness techniques are key to navigating challenges effectively. By acknowledging these special considerations and implementing tailored strategies, individuals can overcome hurdles, maintain motivation, and achieve sustainable weight management and overall well-being.

UNDERSTANDING WEIGHT MANAGEMENT: 2024 EDITION

CHAPTER 7

Weight Management in Children and Adolescents

1. Establishing Healthy Habits

Balanced Nutrition: Emphasize whole foods, fruits, vegetables, and limit sugary snacks to instill healthy eating habits early on.

Physical Activity: Encourage regular exercise and limit screen time to promote an active lifestyle and prevent sedentary behaviors.

2. Family Involvement

Family Meals: Promote family meals and involvement in meal planning to instill healthy eating patterns and foster family bonding.

Positive Role Models: Set positive examples by demonstrating healthy eating habits and engaging in physical activities together.

Weight Management in Young Adults (18-35)

1. Balancing Independence and Health

Nutrition Education: Encourage learning about balanced nutrition and mindful eating to make informed food choices.

Fitness Diversity: Explore various fitness activities to find enjoyable exercises that can be incorporated into a busy lifestyle.

2. Stress Management

Stress Reduction Techniques: Practice stress-reducing activities like yoga, meditation, or mindfulness to avoid stress-induced eating.

Healthy Coping Mechanisms: Develop healthy coping mechanisms to manage stress without resorting to unhealthy eating habits.

Weight Management in Middle-aged Adults (36-60)

1. Metabolism and Hormonal Changes

Metabolism Awareness: Be mindful of slowing metabolism and adjust dietary intake and exercise routines accordingly.

Hormonal Influences: Understand hormonal changes and their impact on weight gain, seeking strategies to mitigate these effects.

2. Lifestyle Modifications

Balanced Diet: Emphasize nutrient-dense foods and portion control to maintain a healthy weight while meeting changing nutritional needs.

Regular Health Screenings: Prioritize regular health check-ups to address any underlying health

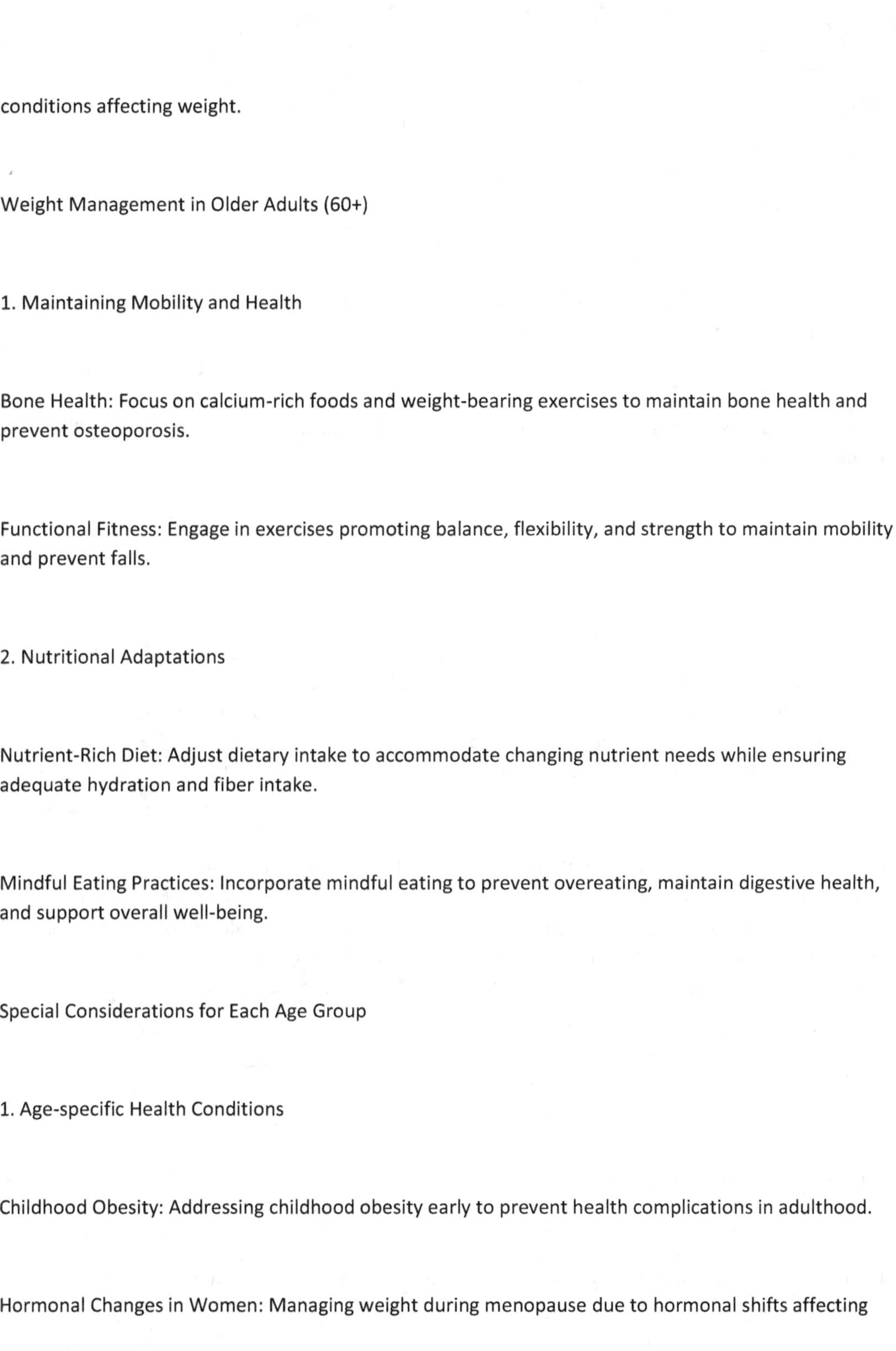

conditions affecting weight.

Weight Management in Older Adults (60+)

1. Maintaining Mobility and Health

Bone Health: Focus on calcium-rich foods and weight-bearing exercises to maintain bone health and prevent osteoporosis.

Functional Fitness: Engage in exercises promoting balance, flexibility, and strength to maintain mobility and prevent falls.

2. Nutritional Adaptations

Nutrient-Rich Diet: Adjust dietary intake to accommodate changing nutrient needs while ensuring adequate hydration and fiber intake.

Mindful Eating Practices: Incorporate mindful eating to prevent overeating, maintain digestive health, and support overall well-being.

Special Considerations for Each Age Group

1. Age-specific Health Conditions

Childhood Obesity: Addressing childhood obesity early to prevent health complications in adulthood.

Hormonal Changes in Women: Managing weight during menopause due to hormonal shifts affecting metabolism.

2. Emotional Well-being

Adolescent Mental Health: Addressing body image concerns and fostering a positive relationship with food and body image.

Senior Isolation: Promoting social engagement and combating isolation to maintain mental well-being and healthy habits.

Conclusion

Weight management strategies should be tailored to the specific needs and considerations of each age group. Encouraging healthy habits from childhood, promoting balanced nutrition, regular exercise, stress management, and adapting to changing physiological and lifestyle factors are crucial across different age demographics. By addressing age-specific challenges and implementing age-appropriate strategies, individuals can achieve and maintain healthy weight management throughout their lifespan.

Weight management strategies for different age groups should consider developmental stages, physiological changes, and lifestyle factors unique to each demographic. Implementing age-appropriate strategies fosters healthy habits early on and adapts to changing needs as individuals progress through different life stages. By addressing these specific considerations, individuals can navigate weight management effectively, ensuring a healthy and balanced lifestyle across various age groups.

Weight Management for Children and Adolescents

1. Promoting Healthy Eating Habits

Nutrient-Rich Diet: Encourage balanced meals with fruits, vegetables, lean proteins, and whole grains to support growth and development.

Limiting Sugary Drinks and Snacks: Discourage excessive consumption of sugary beverages and snacks, promoting healthier alternatives.

2. Encouraging Physical Activity

Active Lifestyle: Advocate for at least 60 minutes of moderate-to-vigorous physical activity daily to enhance cardiovascular health and maintain a healthy weight.

Limiting Screen Time: Encourage a limit on screen time, replacing it with outdoor play, sports, or other physical activities.

Addressing Weight-Related Challenges in Older Adults

1. Maintaining Mobility and Strength

Balance and Flexibility Exercises: Promote exercises like yoga, tai chi, or Pilates to improve balance, flexibility, and reduce the risk of falls.

Strength Training: Encourage resistance exercises to preserve muscle mass, improve metabolism, and maintain functional independence.

2. Nutrition and Health Considerations

Nutrient-Dense Diet: Emphasize calcium-rich foods, lean proteins, and adequate hydration to support bone health and prevent muscle loss.

Regular Health Screenings: Advocate for regular health check-ups to monitor weight-related health conditions and adjust lifestyle accordingly.

Pregnancy, Postpartum Weight, and Weight Management

1. Healthy Weight Gain During Pregnancy

Balanced Nutrition: Encourage a well-balanced diet supporting the nutritional needs of the mother and the developing baby.

Moderate Exercise: Promote safe, low-impact exercises approved by healthcare providers to support maternal health and manage weight gain.

2. Postpartum Weight Management

Gradual Return to Exercise: Encourage gradual resumption of physical activity after childbirth, focusing on postnatal exercises and pelvic floor strengthening.

Balancing Nutrition: Emphasize balanced meals while considering the energy needs of breastfeeding mothers and making healthy food choices.

Special Considerations and Challenges in Each Group

1. Children and Adolescents

Behavioral and Emotional Health: Address body image concerns, foster a positive relationship with food, and educate on the dangers of extreme dieting.

Parental Involvement: Engage parents in promoting healthy habits at home, including meal planning and encouraging physical activities.

2. Older Adults

Chronic Health Conditions: Tailor weight management strategies to accommodate conditions like arthritis, heart disease, or diabetes for safe and effective outcomes.

Social Engagement: Combat social isolation by integrating fitness activities into group settings, fostering camaraderie and motivation.

3. Pregnancy and Postpartum

Breastfeeding Support: Offer guidance on maintaining a nutritious diet while breastfeeding to support both the mother's and baby's health.

Mindful Recovery: Encourage self-compassion and patience post-birth, focusing on gradual weight loss and prioritizing overall well-being.

Conclusion

Weight management strategies differ across age groups due to distinct physiological, developmental, and lifestyle factors. For children and adolescents, emphasizing healthy eating habits and promoting physical activity are fundamental. Older adults benefit from maintaining mobility, strength, and tailored nutrition. During pregnancy and postpartum, focus on balanced nutrition, safe exercises, and gradual weight management. Addressing specific challenges within each demographic ensures age-appropriate and effective weight management strategies, promoting overall health and well-being across different life stages.

Weight management strategies for children, adolescents, older adults, and individuals during pregnancy and postpartum vary significantly due to specific developmental, physiological, and lifestyle factors. Tailoring strategies to each group involves promoting healthy habits, addressing age-specific challenges, and emphasizing a balanced approach to nutrition and exercise. By understanding and addressing the unique needs of each demographic, effective and age-appropriate weight management strategies can be implemented to support overall health and well-being at different stages of life.

Medical Interventions for Weight Control

1. Bariatric Surgery

Gastric Bypass: Surgical procedure that reduces stomach size and reroutes the digestive tract, promoting reduced food intake and nutrient absorption.

Gastric Sleeve: Removes a portion of the stomach, limiting food capacity and reducing hunger-inducing hormones.

Adjustable Gastric Banding: Involves placing a band around the stomach to restrict food intake, creating a feeling of fullness with smaller portions.

2. Pharmacotherapy

Appetite Suppressants: Medications that suppress appetite or induce a feeling of fullness to reduce food intake.

Metabolic Modifiers: Drugs that alter metabolism, aiding in fat breakdown, or reducing absorption of dietary fats.

3. Medical Devices

Intragastric Balloons: Temporary devices inserted into the stomach to occupy space, promoting a feeling of fullness and reduced food intake.

Gastric Electrical Stimulation: Implantable devices that modify stomach contractions to regulate feelings of hunger and satiety.

Effectiveness and Considerations of Medical Interventions

1. Effectiveness of Bariatric Surgery

Weight Loss: Bariatric surgery can lead to substantial weight loss, often resulting in significant improvements in obesity-related health conditions.

Health Benefits: Improvements in diabetes, hypertension, and obstructive sleep apnea are commonly observed post-surgery.

2. Safety and Risks

Surgical Risks: Bariatric surgeries carry risks like infection, blood clots, or nutritional deficiencies, necessitating careful consideration and medical supervision.

Pharmacotherapy Risks: Side effects like increased heart rate, insomnia, or gastrointestinal issues may accompany pharmacological interventions.

Patient Selection and Post-Intervention Care

1. Patient Selection Criteria

BMI and Health Conditions: Patients with a BMI over 40 or with obesity-related health conditions may be candidates for bariatric surgery.

Failed Weight Loss Attempts: Individuals who have attempted traditional weight loss methods without success may consider medical interventions.

2. Post-Intervention Care

Dietary Modifications: Post-surgery or medication, dietary changes are crucial for optimal outcomes, often requiring lifelong adherence to specific guidelines.

Behavioral Support: Psychological counseling or support groups help address emotional aspects, coping mechanisms, and lifestyle changes post-intervention.

Integration with Lifestyle Changes

1. Complementary Lifestyle Modifications

Healthy Eating Patterns: Combined with medical interventions, adopting balanced, nutrient-dense diets enhances weight loss outcomes.

Regular Exercise: Incorporating physical activity post-intervention aids in maintaining weight loss and improving overall health.

2. Long-Term Management

Sustained Follow-ups: Regular medical follow-ups and support are essential for monitoring progress and addressing potential complications.

Behavioral Modifications: Fostering lasting behavioral changes and a positive relationship with food aids in sustaining weight loss achievements.

Ethical Considerations and Future Directions

1. Ethical Considerations

Informed Consent: Ensuring patients have a thorough understanding of risks, benefits, and alternatives before opting for medical interventions.

Equity and Accessibility: Addressing disparities in access to medical interventions and ensuring fair availability for all demographics.

2. Future Research and Advancements

Innovative Approaches: Ongoing research explores less invasive procedures, improved medications, and personalized interventions for better outcomes and reduced risks.

Multidisciplinary Approaches: Collaborative efforts between healthcare professionals, researchers, and policymakers aim to enhance overall care and outcomes for individuals seeking medical interventions for weight control.

Conclusion

Medical interventions play a significant role in weight control for individuals facing challenges in achieving sustainable weight loss through traditional methods. Bariatric surgeries, pharmacotherapy, and medical devices offer viable options with varying degrees of effectiveness and risks. Patient selection, post-intervention care, integration with lifestyle modifications, and ethical considerations are crucial factors for successful outcomes. Advancements in research and multidisciplinary approaches continue to shape the landscape of medical interventions, aiming for improved effectiveness, safety, and accessibility in weight control.

Medical interventions like bariatric surgery, pharmacotherapy, and medical devices provide viable options for individuals facing challenges in achieving weight control through traditional means. These interventions come with varying degrees of effectiveness, risks, and ethical considerations. Integrating medical interventions with lifestyle modifications and long-term management strategies are crucial for successful outcomes. Ongoing research and advancements aim to enhance the effectiveness, safety, and accessibility of medical interventions for weight control, offering hope for improved outcomes and better quality of life for individuals seeking these treatments.

Exploring Medical Options for Weight Loss

1. Understanding Medical Interventions

Bariatric Surgery: Invasive procedures altering the digestive system's anatomy to induce weight loss.

Pharmacotherapy: Medications targeting appetite suppression, altering metabolism, or reducing fat absorption to aid weight loss.

2. Considerations and Effectiveness

Patient Selection Criteria: Evaluation based on BMI, obesity-related health conditions, failed weight loss attempts through traditional means, and risk assessment.

Effectiveness: Variable effectiveness among individuals, with factors like adherence, lifestyle modifications, and physiological responses influencing outcomes.

Bariatric Surgery and Its Role in Weight Management

1. Types of Bariatric Surgery

Gastric Bypass: Restructuring the digestive system by creating a smaller stomach pouch and bypassing a portion of the small intestine.

Gastric Sleeve: Surgical removal of a portion of the stomach to limit food intake and regulate hunger hormones.

Adjustable Gastric Banding: Placing a band around the upper part of the stomach to create a smaller pouch, restricting food intake.

2. Effectiveness and Benefits

Substantial Weight Loss: Bariatric surgery often leads to significant weight loss, resulting in improvements in obesity-related health conditions like diabetes and hypertension.

Metabolic Changes: Alterations in gut hormones and metabolic processes contribute to reduced hunger and improved weight control.

Medications and Their Effectiveness in Weight Control

1. Types of Weight Loss Medications

Appetite Suppressants: Targeting hunger-regulating hormones or neurotransmitters to reduce appetite.

Metabolic Modifiers: Drugs affecting metabolism, facilitating fat breakdown, or reducing nutrient absorption.

2. Effectiveness and Considerations

Varied Response: Efficacy differs among individuals, influenced by factors like adherence, side effects, and individual physiological responses.

Adverse Effects: Side effects may include increased heart rate, insomnia, gastrointestinal disturbances, or potential dependency, necessitating careful monitoring.

Patient Selection and Monitoring

1. Patient Eligibility and Considerations

Criteria for Medication Use: Evaluation based on BMI, obesity-related health conditions, previous weight loss attempts, and medical history.

Psychological and Behavioral Factors: Addressing emotional eating, mental health concerns, and behavioral patterns affecting weight control.

2. Monitoring and Follow-Up Care

Lifestyle Modifications: Integration with healthy eating habits, regular exercise, and behavioral changes to optimize outcomes.

Regular Follow-Ups: Monitoring progress, addressing concerns, adjusting medications, and providing ongoing support for sustained weight loss.

Safety, Risks, and Ethical Considerations

1. Safety and Risks

Surgical Risks: Potential complications like infection, blood clots, nutritional deficiencies, and long-term anatomical changes.

Medication Risks: Side effects, drug interactions, and potential health risks requiring vigilant monitoring and management.

2. Ethical Considerations

Informed Consent: Ensuring patients understand risks, benefits, and alternatives before choosing medical interventions.

Equity and Accessibility: Addressing disparities in access to medical options and ensuring fair availability across demographics.

Conclusion

Exploring medical options for weight loss encompasses bariatric surgery and pharmacotherapy, each with its effectiveness, considerations, and risks. Bariatric surgery offers substantial weight loss and health benefits but involves surgical risks and long-term anatomical changes. Weight loss medications, while offering options, present varying effectiveness and potential adverse effects. Patient selection, careful monitoring, lifestyle modifications, and ethical considerations are crucial for optimal outcomes. Balancing the benefits and risks, tailoring interventions to individual needs, and ensuring informed decisions form the cornerstone of effective medical options for weight loss.

Medical options for weight loss, including bariatric surgery and medications, provide viable approaches but come with considerations and risks. Bariatric surgery offers substantial weight loss and health benefits but entails surgical risks and long-term anatomical changes. Weight loss medications, though available, exhibit varying effectiveness and potential adverse effects. Patient selection, monitoring, lifestyle modifications, and ethical considerations are critical for successful outcomes. Personalized interventions, informed decisions, and a balanced assessment of benefits versus risks are key in utilizing medical options for weight loss effectively.

UNDERSTANDING WEIGHT MANAGEMENT: 2024 EDITION

CHAPTER 8

The Role of Social Support in Weight Management

1. Emotional Support

Encouragement: Positive reinforcement and encouragement from friends, family, or support groups foster motivation and adherence to healthy habits.

Understanding and Empathy: Having a supportive network that understands the challenges aids in navigating setbacks and staying resilient.

2. Accountability and Motivation

Accountability Partners: Sharing goals and progress with others creates a sense of accountability, motivating individuals to stay on track.

Healthy Competition: Friendly competitions or challenges within a social circle can motivate individuals to achieve their weight management goals.

Community Engagement for Weight Management

1. Support Groups and Programs

Peer Support Networks: Joining weight loss groups or programs offers camaraderie, shared experiences, and valuable tips for success.

Online Communities: Engaging in online forums or social media groups provides access to a broader community, offering advice and motivation.

2. Community-based Interventions

Local Initiatives: Participating in community-based wellness events, workshops, or fitness classes fosters a sense of belonging and promotes healthy habits.

Collaborative Efforts: Partnering with local organizations or health professionals encourages collective efforts in promoting healthy living within the community.

Benefits of Social Support and Community Engagement

1. Enhanced Adherence and Consistency

Consistent Motivation: Social support provides consistent motivation, reducing the likelihood of giving up on weight management goals.

Adherence to Healthy Behaviors: Being part of a supportive environment encourages adherence to healthier eating habits and regular exercise routines.

2. Psychological Well-being

Reduced Stress: Social connections alleviate stress, lowering the likelihood of stress-induced overeating or unhealthy coping mechanisms.

Improved Self-esteem: Positive social interactions boost self-confidence and self-worth, contributing to a positive body image.

Challenges and Strategies for Effective Support

1. Challenges in Social Support

Unsupportive Environments: Lack of support or encountering negative influences can hinder progress and motivation.

Over-reliance: Dependency on social support without fostering self-motivation might impede personal progress.

2. Strategies for Effective Support

Open Communication: Clear communication of needs and expectations fosters better support within social circles.

Diverse Support Networks: Building diverse support networks ensures access to varied perspectives and resources.

Integration of Social Support into Weight Management Plans

1. Incorporating Support Mechanisms

Family Involvement: Engaging family members in meal planning, activities, and discussions about healthy habits creates a supportive home environment.

Peer Support Systems: Joining or forming groups with similar weight management goals encourages mutual support and accountability.

2. Utilizing Technology

Mobile Apps and Online Tools: Utilizing apps or online platforms for tracking progress and connecting with support communities.

Virtual Support Networks: Virtual meet-ups or support groups offer accessibility and engagement for individuals unable to access in-person communities.

Conclusion

Social support and community engagement play pivotal roles in successful weight management by providing motivation, accountability, and emotional reinforcement. Access to supportive networks, participation in community programs, and leveraging diverse resources create an environment conducive to sustaining healthy lifestyle changes. Despite challenges, integrating social support into weight management plans empowers individuals to navigate obstacles and achieve long-term success.

By fostering supportive relationships and active community engagement, individuals can effectively maintain healthy behaviors and achieve their weight management goals.

Social support and community engagement are crucial elements in successful weight management, providing motivation, accountability, and emotional reinforcement. Access to supportive networks, participation in community programs, and leveraging diverse resources create an environment conducive to sustaining healthy lifestyle changes. Despite challenges, integrating social support into weight management plans empowers individuals to navigate obstacles and achieve long-term success. By fostering supportive relationships and active community engagement, individuals can effectively maintain healthy behaviors and achieve their weight management goals.

Understanding Support Systems

1. Defining Support Systems

Social Networks: Family, friends, colleagues, mentors, and communities that offer guidance, encouragement, and assistance.

Types of Support: Emotional support, informational support, instrumental support, and appraisal support.

2. Roles of Support Systems

Emotional Reinforcement: Providing comfort, empathy, and encouragement during challenging times, reducing stress and anxiety.

Resource Access: Offering access to knowledge, resources, and guidance for decision-making and problem-solving.

Health and Well-being Benefits of Support Systems

1. Mental Health Support

Stress Reduction: Supportive networks alleviate stress, promoting better mental health and reducing the risk of depression or anxiety.

Coping Mechanisms: Providing coping strategies and outlets, enhancing resilience in dealing with life's challenges.

2. Physical Health Benefits

Healthier Habits: Encouragement from support systems promotes healthy behaviors like exercise, proper nutrition, and regular health check-ups.

Faster Recovery: Support systems aid in recovery from illnesses or medical treatments, positively impacting healing processes.

Impact on Personal Growth and Development

1. Encouragement for Goals

Motivation: Supportive networks offer motivation, boosting confidence and determination in pursuing personal and professional goals.

Constructive Feedback: Honest feedback and guidance from support systems facilitate learning and growth.

2. Enhancing Skills and Knowledge

Skill Building: Opportunities within support systems foster skill development through mentorship, workshops, or learning communities.

Access to Information: Sharing of experiences and knowledge expands perspectives, aiding in informed decision-making.

Professional Success and Career Advancement

1. Networking and Opportunities

Career Guidance: Support networks offer career advice, networking opportunities, and mentorship, aiding in career progression.

Access to Opportunities: Recommendations or referrals from supportive contacts enhance access to job opportunities or professional growth.

2. Workplace Support

Workplace Environment: Supportive colleagues and supervisors foster a positive work environment, enhancing job satisfaction and productivity.

Conflict Resolution: Support systems aid in conflict resolution and problem-solving within the workplace.

Navigating Life Transitions and Challenges

1. Support During Life Changes

Transition Support: During major life events like relocation, relationship changes, or personal milestones, supportive networks offer guidance and comfort.

Financial Support: Assistance during financial difficulties or uncertainties aids in managing challenges effectively.

2. Resilience and Adaptability

Building Resilience: Support systems contribute to building resilience, enabling individuals to bounce back from setbacks or failures.

Adaptability: Assistance and advice during changes or crises aid in adapting to new circumstances more effectively.

Cultivating Support Systems

1. Building and Maintaining Relationships

Mutual Support: Nurturing relationships through reciprocity ensures a two-way supportive dynamic.

Open Communication: Effective communication fosters deeper connections and understanding within support networks.

2. Diverse Support Networks

Diversity in Networks: Having varied support networks ensures access to different perspectives, resources, and opportunities.

Balancing Dependence and Independence: Maintaining a balance between self-reliance and seeking help when needed fosters healthy relationships.

Conclusion

Support systems play multifaceted roles in individuals' lives, impacting health, personal growth, career advancement, and resilience during life's challenges. Emotional reinforcement, resource access, and guidance from support networks significantly contribute to overall well-being and success. Cultivating diverse and nurturing relationships while maintaining a balance between independence and seeking help when necessary is crucial for harnessing the benefits of support systems. Recognizing the significance of supportive networks and actively fostering these connections can positively influence various aspects of life, ensuring a more fulfilling and resilient journey.

Support systems play multifaceted roles in individuals' lives, impacting health, personal growth, career advancement, and resilience during life's challenges. Emotional reinforcement, resource access, and guidance from support networks significantly contribute to overall well-being and success. Cultivating diverse and nurturing relationships while maintaining a balance between independence and seeking help when necessary is crucial for harnessing the benefits of support systems. Recognizing the significance of supportive networks and actively fostering these connections can positively influence various aspects of life, ensuring a more fulfilling and resilient journey.

The Role of Family and Friends in Weight Management

1. Emotional Support and Encouragement

Motivational Influence: Family and friends can serve as motivators, providing encouragement and positive reinforcement towards weight loss goals.

Accountability: Involving loved ones creates a sense of accountability, fostering commitment to healthier habits.

2. Lifestyle Adaptations

Shared Healthy Habits: Engaging in activities such as meal planning, exercising together, or adopting healthier recipes as a family unit promotes collective wellness.

Influence on Environment: Creating supportive environments at home, with healthier food choices readily available, facilitates weight management.

Finding Community Support for Weight Loss Goals

1. Joining Support Groups and Programs

Local Support Groups: Participating in community-based weight loss programs or support groups offers encouragement and shared experiences.

Fitness Classes or Clubs: Engaging in group fitness activities fosters camaraderie and mutual support.

2. Utilizing Community Resources

Community Centers: Accessing resources like nutrition workshops, cooking classes, or fitness sessions provided by local community centers promotes healthy habits.

Volunteer Organizations: Joining volunteer groups engaged in wellness initiatives not only supports the community but also provides a supportive network.

Online Resources and Communities for Weight Management

1. Online Support Networks

Social Media Groups: Engaging in online communities dedicated to weight management allows sharing experiences, tips, and encouragement.

Fitness Apps and Websites: Utilizing apps and websites offering fitness tracking, meal planning, and motivational content facilitates adherence to weight management goals.

2. Professional Online Guidance

Telemedicine and Virtual Support: Accessing telehealth services for consultations, personalized advice, or virtual support from nutritionists and fitness coaches.

Webinars and Forums: Participating in online webinars, forums, or Q&A sessions with experts provides valuable insights and guidance.

Benefits of Family, Friends, Community, and Online Support

1. Motivation and Accountability

Continuous Encouragement: Support networks provide ongoing motivation, celebrating successes and offering encouragement during setbacks.

Shared Experiences: Sharing experiences with others on a similar journey creates a sense of solidarity and encouragement to stay focused.

2. Access to Resources and Information

Information Sharing: Accessing diverse perspectives and information through support networks broadens knowledge on effective weight management strategies.

Resource Pooling: Shared resources within communities or online forums offer a wealth of tips, recipes, and exercise routines.

Addressing Challenges and Maximizing Benefits

1. Overcoming Resistance and Conflicts

Communication and Understanding: Open dialogue and understanding among family and friends alleviate resistance and potential conflicts regarding lifestyle changes.

Building Consensus: Consensus-building within communities or online groups fosters a shared commitment to wellness goals.

2. Critical Evaluation of Online Resources

Reliability Check: Verifying the credibility of online information and advice ensures following evidence-based strategies.

Balancing Online Engagement: Moderating online interactions to avoid information overload or detrimental comparisons.

Conclusion

The involvement of family, friends, engagement within community networks, and utilization of online resources significantly impact successful weight management. Support from loved ones offers emotional reinforcement and encouragement, fostering commitment and accountability. Community engagement provides a sense of belonging and shared experiences, while online resources offer diverse perspectives and access to information. Addressing challenges and maximizing the benefits of these support systems involve effective communication, critical evaluation of resources, and a balanced approach to engagement. By leveraging the collective support from family, friends, communities, and online platforms, individuals can enhance their journey towards sustainable weight management.

The involvement of family, friends, community engagement, and utilization of online resources significantly impacts successful weight management. Support from loved ones offers emotional reinforcement and encouragement, fostering commitment and accountability. Community engagement provides a sense of belonging and shared experiences, while online resources offer diverse perspectives and access to information. Addressing challenges and maximizing the benefits of these support systems involve effective communication, critical evaluation of resources, and a balanced approach to engagement. By leveraging the collective support from family, friends, communities, and online platforms, individuals can enhance their journey towards sustainable weight management.

Technological Advancements in Weight Management

1. Digital Health Solutions

Advanced Tracking Devices: Integration of wearables and smart devices offering enhanced accuracy in monitoring physical activity, sleep, and dietary habits.

AI-Powered Apps: Utilizing artificial intelligence for personalized recommendations, meal planning, and real-time coaching based on individual data.

2. Telehealth and Virtual Support

Remote Consultations: Increasing accessibility to nutritionists, dietitians, and fitness experts through telehealth services for personalized guidance.

Virtual Support Communities: Enhanced online platforms offering immersive experiences and real-time support for individuals seeking community engagement.

Innovations in Nutrition and Dietary Approaches

1. Personalized Nutrition

Nutrigenomics: Tailoring diets based on an individual's genetic makeup to optimize weight management and overall health.

Precision Nutrition: Advanced algorithms analyzing individual biomarkers, microbiome data, and lifestyle factors to create customized dietary plans.

2. Functional Foods and Supplements

Nutrient-Dense Innovations: Development of functional foods providing concentrated nutrients, aiding in weight management and overall health.

Targeted Supplements: Customized supplements targeting specific deficiencies or metabolic functions for improved weight control.

Advancements in Fitness and Physical Activity

1. Virtual Fitness Experiences

Virtual Reality Workouts: Immersive fitness experiences through VR technology, offering engaging and interactive exercise routines.

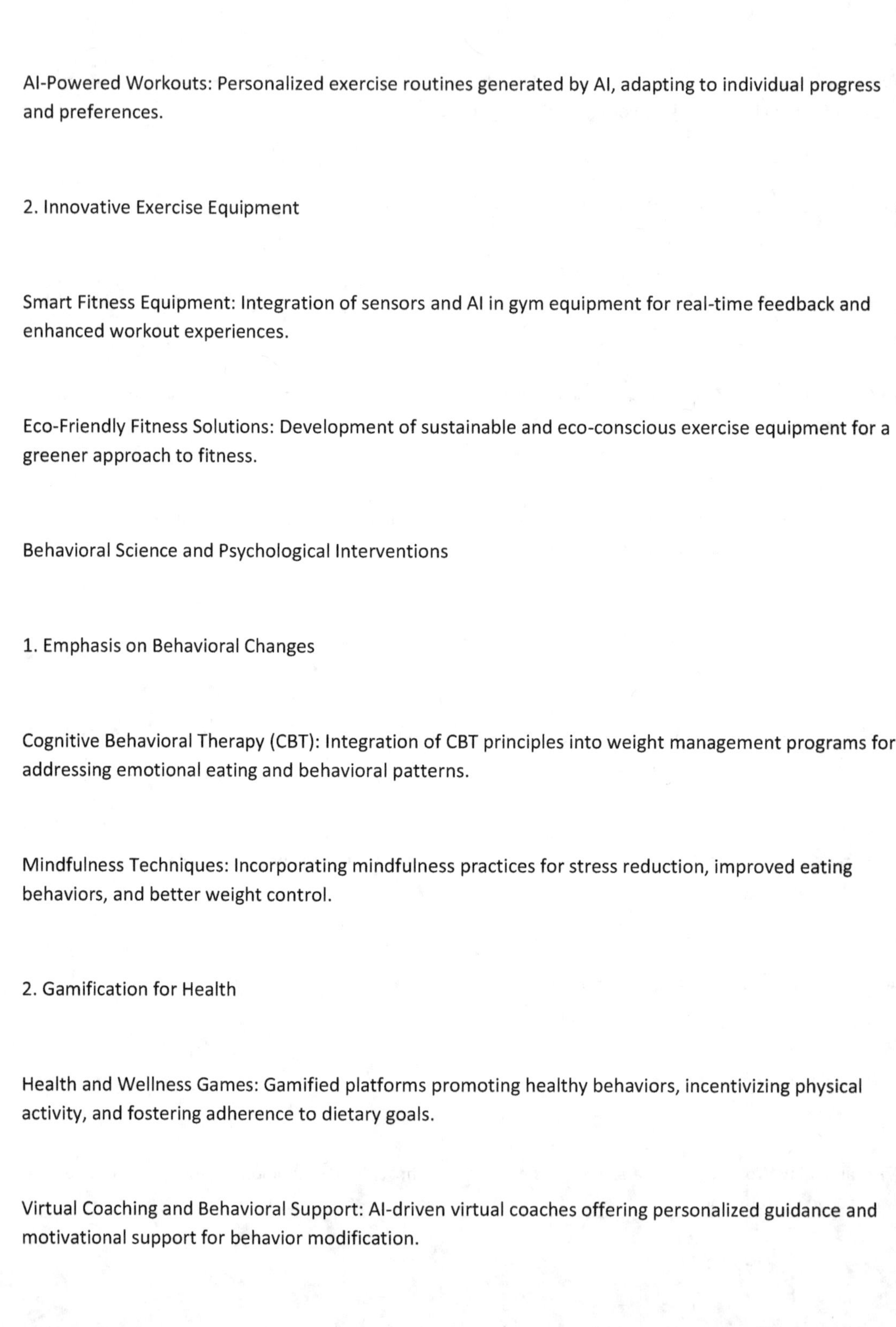

AI-Powered Workouts: Personalized exercise routines generated by AI, adapting to individual progress and preferences.

2. Innovative Exercise Equipment

Smart Fitness Equipment: Integration of sensors and AI in gym equipment for real-time feedback and enhanced workout experiences.

Eco-Friendly Fitness Solutions: Development of sustainable and eco-conscious exercise equipment for a greener approach to fitness.

Behavioral Science and Psychological Interventions

1. Emphasis on Behavioral Changes

Cognitive Behavioral Therapy (CBT): Integration of CBT principles into weight management programs for addressing emotional eating and behavioral patterns.

Mindfulness Techniques: Incorporating mindfulness practices for stress reduction, improved eating behaviors, and better weight control.

2. Gamification for Health

Health and Wellness Games: Gamified platforms promoting healthy behaviors, incentivizing physical activity, and fostering adherence to dietary goals.

Virtual Coaching and Behavioral Support: AI-driven virtual coaches offering personalized guidance and motivational support for behavior modification.

Environmental and Societal Influences

1. Focus on Sustainable Practices

Environmental Impact Consideration: Integration of sustainable practices in weight management programs, promoting eco-friendly approaches.

Social Responsibility: Addressing societal influences like food deserts or accessibility issues, ensuring equitable access to health resources.

2. Cultural Sensitivity and Inclusivity

Diverse Representation: Tailoring programs considering diverse cultural backgrounds, preferences, and dietary habits for inclusivity.

Community-Centric Approaches: Collaborative efforts involving local communities for culturally relevant and sustainable health initiatives.

Conclusion

The future of weight management is poised for revolutionary advancements, encompassing technological innovations, personalized approaches, behavioral interventions, and societal considerations. From AI-driven personalized nutrition to virtual fitness experiences and sustainable health practices, future trends promise enhanced accessibility, customization, and effectiveness in weight management. Integrating advancements in technology, nutrition, fitness, behavioral sciences, and cultural sensitivity ensures a holistic and personalized approach to empower individuals on their journey towards healthier lifestyles and sustainable weight control.

The future of weight management is poised for revolutionary advancements, encompassing technological innovations, personalized approaches, behavioral interventions, and societal considerations. From AI-driven personalized nutrition to virtual fitness experiences and sustainable health practices, future trends promise enhanced accessibility, customization, and effectiveness in weight management. Integrating advancements in technology, nutrition, fitness, behavioral sciences, and cultural sensitivity ensures a holistic and personalized approach to empower individuals on their journey towards healthier lifestyles and sustainable weight control.

UNDERSTANDING WEIGHT MANAGEMENT: 2024 EDITION

CHAPTER 9

Wearable Devices and Health Trackers

1. Advanced Health Monitoring

Biometric Sensors: Wearable devices integrating advanced sensors for precise tracking of vital signs, physical activity, and sleep patterns.

Continuous Data Collection: Real-time monitoring of heart rate variability, stress levels, and calorie expenditure for personalized insights.

2. AI-Powered Health Insights

Machine Learning Algorithms: Analyzing extensive data sets to provide predictive analytics and personalized recommendations for diet and exercise.

Behavioral Feedback: AI-generated insights assisting users in making informed decisions and modifying behaviors for better weight management.

Telemedicine and Remote Coaching

1. Virtual Consultations

Remote Healthcare Services: Access to nutritionists, dietitians, and fitness coaches through telemedicine for tailored guidance and support.

Continuous Remote Monitoring: Utilizing wearable devices to transmit health data, enabling real-time adjustments to weight management strategies.

2. AI-Powered Virtual Coaches

Personalized Coaching: AI-driven virtual coaches offering customized exercise routines, dietary suggestions, and motivational support.

Behavioral Modification: AI interventions providing behavioral coaching for habit formation and adherence to weight management plans.

Precision Nutrition and Genetic Insights

1. Genetic Testing for Personalized Nutrition

Nutrigenomics: Analyzing genetic data to design tailored dietary plans based on an individual's genetic predispositions.

Microbiome Analysis: Understanding gut microbiota to recommend personalized diets promoting weight loss and overall health.

2. Smart Nutritional Solutions

Meal Replacement Innovations: Customized meal replacement options with precise nutrient compositions for weight control and dietary adherence.

Nutrient-Dense Foods: Development of nutrient-dense food products catering to specific nutritional needs for improved weight management.

Virtual Reality (VR) and Immersive Fitness

1. Immersive Fitness Experiences

Virtual Workout Sessions: VR technology offering immersive fitness experiences with interactive workouts and gamified training routines.

Personalized Fitness Environments: Customizable VR settings catering to individual preferences for enhanced engagement and motivation.

2. VR for Behavioral Modification

Exposure Therapy: VR-based interventions for combating food cravings, stress management, and behavioral modifications aiding weight control.

Mindfulness and Stress Reduction: Immersive VR experiences facilitating relaxation, stress reduction, and mindful eating practices.

Artificial Intelligence in Behavioral Modification

1. Cognitive Behavioral Therapy (CBT) Integration

Cognitive Training: AI-powered apps integrating CBT principles for addressing emotional eating, stress management, and behavior modification.

Mental Health Support: AI-driven interventions providing mental health resources and coping strategies for effective weight management.

2. Behavioral Gamification for Motivation

Health and Wellness Games: Gamified platforms using AI to foster motivation, adherence to fitness routines, and healthy eating habits.

Virtual Coaching and Support: AI-driven virtual coaches providing continuous guidance and motivation to facilitate behavior change.

Conclusion

Emerging technologies in weight management encompass wearables, AI-driven solutions, precision nutrition, immersive fitness experiences, and behavioral modification tools. These innovations offer personalized, data-driven approaches to support individuals in their weight management journey. Integrating advanced technologies, telemedicine, genetic insights, and immersive experiences ensures tailored strategies promoting adherence, motivation, and long-term success in weight control. The future of weight management is evolving with a focus on customization, accessibility, and behavioral modification, empowering individuals to achieve healthier lifestyles and sustainable weight goals.

Emerging technologies in weight management encompass wearables, AI-driven solutions, precision nutrition, immersive fitness experiences, and behavioral modification tools. These innovations offer personalized, data-driven approaches to support individuals in their weight management journey. Integrating advanced technologies, telemedicine, genetic insights, and immersive experiences ensures tailored strategies promoting adherence, motivation, and long-term success in weight control. The future of weight management is evolving with a focus on customization, accessibility, and behavioral modification, empowering individuals to achieve healthier lifestyles and sustainable weight goals.

Wearable Devices and Weight Control

1. Tracking Physical Activity and Exercise

Activity Monitors: Wearables track steps, distance, and calories burned, encouraging increased physical activity for better weight management.

Heart Rate Monitoring: Real-time monitoring provides insights into exercise intensity, aiding in optimizing workouts for weight loss.

2. Monitoring Sleep and Stress

Sleep Tracking: Understanding sleep patterns assists in optimizing rest for improved metabolism and better weight control.

Stress Management: Some wearables track stress levels, encouraging mindfulness and stress reduction, vital for weight management.

Impact of Wearables on Behavior and Motivation

1. Enhancing Accountability and Awareness

Behavioral Modifications: Wearables promote accountability, encouraging users to adopt healthier habits like regular exercise and better sleep.

Self-awareness: Constant tracking fosters self-awareness regarding lifestyle choices, fostering behavioral changes for weight control.

2. Motivational Support

Real-time Feedback: Instant feedback on activity levels motivates users to achieve daily goals, contributing to sustained weight management efforts.

Social Integration: Sharing progress with friends or social networks through wearables fosters a supportive environment, enhancing motivation.

AI and Personalized Weight Management Solutions

1. AI-Driven Nutrition Guidance

Personalized Dietary Plans: AI analyzes individual data to offer tailored meal plans and nutritional recommendations for weight loss goals.

Behavioral Analysis: AI identifies patterns and habits, providing insights for behavioral modifications essential for sustained weight control.

2. Predictive Analytics for Weight Management

Predicting Weight Trends: AI algorithms forecast weight fluctuations based on lifestyle changes, aiding in proactive adjustments to prevent setbacks.

Risk Prediction: Identifying potential health risks related to weight changes enables preemptive measures, promoting overall health.

Future Trends in Weight Management

1. Integration of Wearable AI Solutions

Combined Data Analysis: Integration of wearable data with AI platforms for comprehensive insights into health and weight management.

Health Prediction Models: Advanced predictive models utilizing wearable data to forecast individual health trajectories, facilitating proactive interventions.

2. Personalized Precision Health

Individualized Treatment Plans: Precision health approaches using genetic data and wearables to tailor treatments for weight-related conditions.

Microbiome Analysis: Utilizing wearables to collect data for analyzing gut health and its impact on weight management for personalized strategies.

Ethical and Privacy Considerations

1. Data Privacy and Security

Data Protection: Ensuring user data collected by wearables and AI solutions are securely stored and ethically used for health insights.

Informed Consent: Transparent communication about data usage and the importance of user consent for data sharing and analysis.

2. Equitable Access and Representation

Accessibility: Ensuring affordability and accessibility of wearable devices and AI-driven solutions for diverse populations.

Cultural Sensitivity: Designing inclusive technologies considering diverse cultural backgrounds and preferences for effective weight management.

Conclusion

Wearable devices and AI-driven solutions play a significant role in weight management by tracking physical activity, offering personalized guidance, and motivating behavioral changes. Wearables promote accountability, increase awareness, and offer real-time feedback, crucial for sustaining weight control efforts. AI solutions analyze data for tailored nutrition plans, predict weight trends, and predict health risks. The future of weight management involves integrated wearable AI solutions, personalized precision health approaches, and ethical considerations surrounding data privacy and accessibility. Leveraging advancements in wearables, AI, and personalized health holds promise for more effective, personalized, and accessible weight management solutions, empowering individuals to achieve healthier lifestyles.

Wearable devices and AI-driven solutions significantly impact weight management by tracking physical activity, offering personalized guidance, and motivating behavioral changes. Wearables promote accountability, increase awareness, and offer real-time feedback, crucial for sustaining weight control efforts. AI solutions analyze data for tailored nutrition plans, predict weight trends, and identify health risks. The future of weight management involves integrated wearable AI solutions, personalized precision health approaches, and ethical considerations surrounding data privacy and accessibility. Leveraging advancements in wearables, AI, and personalized health holds promise for more effective, personalized, and accessible weight management solutions, empowering individuals to achieve healthier lifestyles.

UNDERSTANDING WEIGHT MANAGEMENT: 2024 EDITION

CONCLUSION

This book provides a structured approach to cover various aspects of modern weight management, including scientific principles, dietary strategies, exercise, lifestyle changes, special considerations, and future trends. Each chapter could delve deeper into subtopics, providing practical advice, case studies, expert interviews, and actionable steps for readers seeking effective and innovative weight management techniques.